HELLO MUSHROOM COOKBOOK

Mushrooms Made Easy

By

Lucia Johnson-Flores

Hello Mushroom Cookbook

Mushrooms Made Easy

by

Lucia Johnson-Flores

Copyright © 2024

Happy Tales, LLC

www.happytales.biz

PO Box 390428

Edina, MN 55439

ISBN:978-1-965256-09-1 (Paperback)

ISBN: 978-1-965256-10-7 (Hardcover)

ISBN: 978-1-965256-11-4 (Digital)

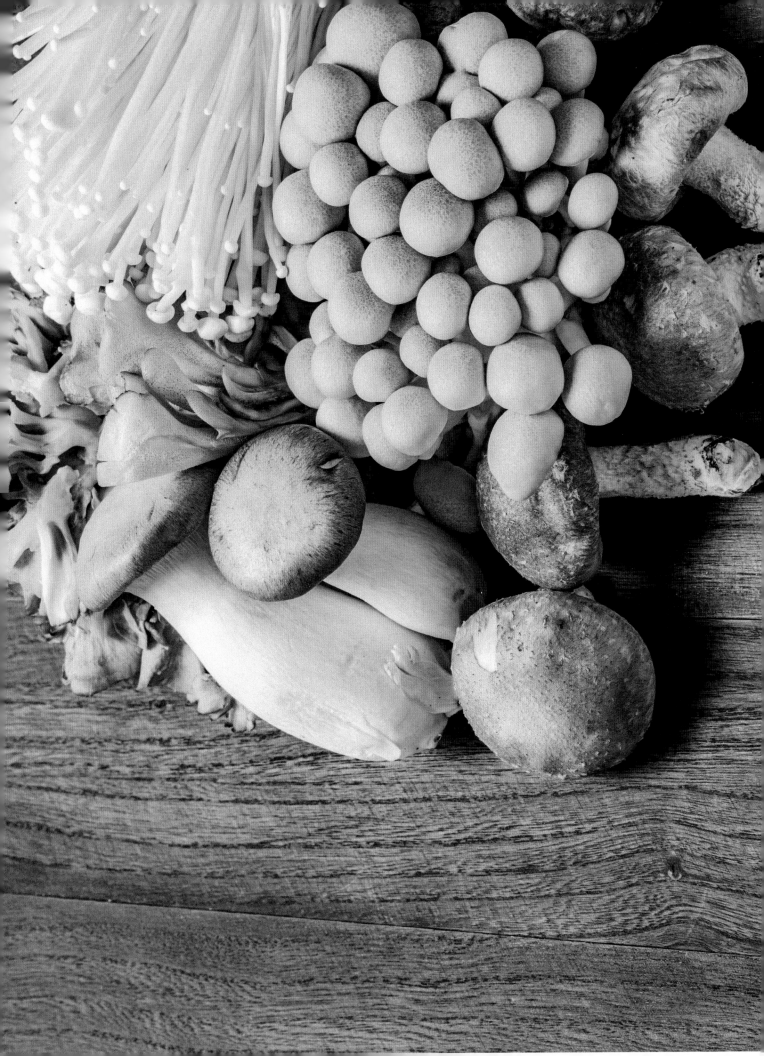

Welcome to the "Hello Mushroom Cookbook." I'm Lucia, and it's my pleasure to share with you my love for one of nature's most fascinating ingredients—mushrooms.

Mushrooms have sparked my imagination and broadened my culinary options. Their diverse textures, rich flavors, and significant health benefits make them a standout addition to any meal. Over the last year, my husband and I have immersed ourselves in the study of various mushroom species, their cultivation methods, and their incredible culinary uses.

In this book, you'll find a collection of my favorite, straightforward recipes that truly demonstrate the adaptability of mushrooms. Whether it's a robust breakfast, a flavorful appetizer, or a comforting soup or main dish, each recipe is crafted to showcase the unique characteristics of mushrooms. I hope these dishes will encourage you to experiment with mushrooms in your kitchen and discover their magical properties.

Thank you for joining me on this gastronomic journey. Let's embark on this exploration into the wonderful world of mushrooms and cook up some delightful meals together.

Lucia

Table of Contents

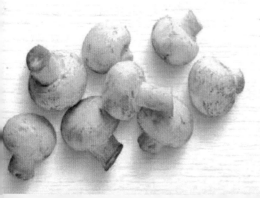

Appetizers 41

Main Dishes 50

Specialty Mushrooms 59

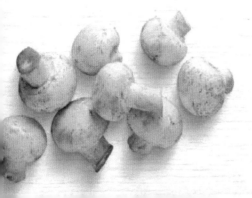

BASICS OF MUSHROOMS

Introduction

Mushrooms hold a special place in cooking traditions around the world. Mushrooms have been used since ancient times and celebrated for their distinctive flavors, textures, and versatility. Mushrooms have really grown to become staples of the culinary arts. Their ability to enhance flavors and their range—from earthy and meaty to delicate and subtle—allows for innovative and delectable cooking.

Historically, mushrooms have been valued not only for their taste but also for their health improving properties. Mushrooms have been used in the traditional medicine for various cultures. Their taste and health benefits have elevated mushrooms from something you might forage for to a highly sought-after ingredient that can transform your meals.

As we learn more about mushrooms and their benefits, they are really going through a revival in the world of food and health supplements. Not only are they a superfood, but they are also sustainable and environmentally friendly. In this cookbook, we will explore different simple recipes to highlight how mushrooms have become unique and essential ingredients that can improve any dish.

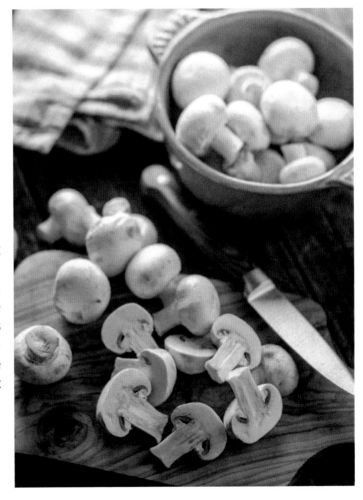

MAIN TYPES OF EDIBLE MUSHROOMS

White Button Mushrooms
(Agaricus bisporus)

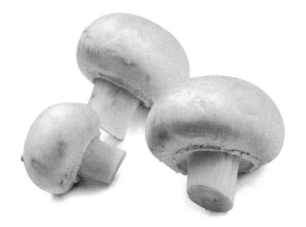

Description:
White button mushrooms are the most common variety of mushroom consumed worldwide. Characterized by their small, round, white caps and short stems, they are harvested early in their growth, before the mushroom cap has fully opened. Their flavor is mild when raw and more earthy when cooked, which makes them highly versatile in the kitchen.

Common Culinary Uses:
White button mushrooms are able to be used in a vast array of dishes. They can be eaten raw in salads or on pizzas for a crisp, mild flavor. When cooked, they develop a more robust taste and can be sautéed, grilled, roasted, or stewed. They are often used in soups, stir-fries, and as an essential ingredient in many sauces. The way they absorb liquid makes them excellent at soaking up flavors from other ingredients, enhancing and complementing the overall dish.

Portobello Mushrooms

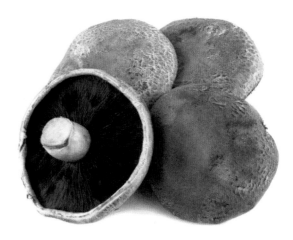

Description:
Portobello mushrooms are mature, brown Agaricus bisporus, closely related to white button mushrooms but larger and with a more developed flavor. They have a broad, flat cap up to 6 inches in diameter with a dense, chewy texture. The deep, meat-like texture and flavor of portobellos make them popular in vegetarian cuisine.

Common Culinary Uses:
Portobello mushrooms are best known for their meatiness and flavor, which makes them perfect for grilling and roasting. Commonly used as a meat substitute in burgers, they can also be stuffed with a variety of ingredients like cheese, herbs, and other vegetables. Sliced portobellos are excellent sautéed and added to pasta dishes, rice and risottos, or served as a side dish.

Chestnut Mushrooms

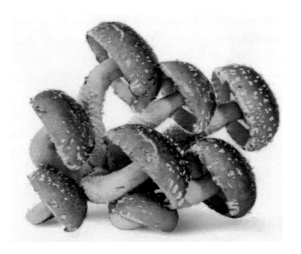

Description:
Chestnut mushrooms are a variant of the white button mushrooms but have a darker, tawny color. They offer a firmer texture and a nuttier, richer flavor than their white counterparts.
Common Culinary Uses:
Versatile in use, chestnut mushrooms can be cooked in similar ways to white mushrooms but are particularly good in recipes where their robust flavor can stand out, such as in stews, sautéed dishes, and as part of a hearty breakfast.

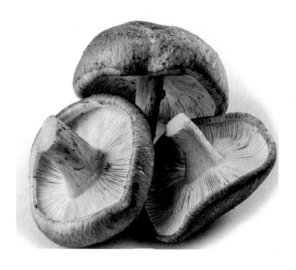

Shiitake Mushrooms

Description:
Shiitake mushrooms are recognized by their umbrella-shaped, slightly curled brown caps, which range from 2 to 4 inches in diameter. They have a rich, earthy flavor and a distinctive aroma that can enhance the flavor profile of many dishes.

Common Culinary Uses:
Shiitakes are extensively used in Asian cuisine, particularly in soups, stir-fries, and broths. They are valued for their umami flavor, making them an excellent addition to vegetarian and meat dishes alike. When dried, shiitakes intensify in flavor and are often rehydrated and added to dishes to impart a deep, savory element.

Lion's Mane Mushrooms

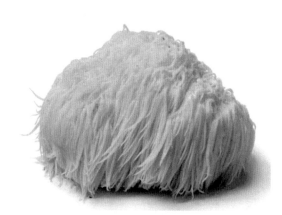

Description:
Lion's Mane mushrooms are distinguished by their unique, shaggy appearance that resembles a white pom pom. This mushroom is noted not only for its striking look but also for its mild, seafood-like flavor.

Common Culinary Uses:
Often used as a substitute for seafood, Lion's Mane can be used in dishes where you might find crab or lobster, such as crab cakes or seafood pasta. It's also delicious when sautéed with butter and garlic, served on toast, or used in soups and sauces.

Oyster Mushrooms (Golden/Brown/White)

Description and Common Culinary Uses:

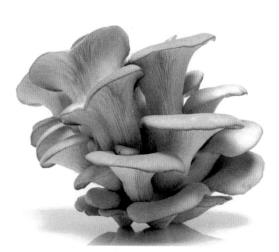

- **Golden Oyster Mushrooms:** Known for their vibrant yellow color, they have a delicate texture and a mild, sweet flavor. They are fantastic in stir-fries or simply sautéed.
- **Brown Oyster Mushrooms:** These mushrooms have a more robust flavor and are excellent in soups and sauces, or grilled.
- **White Oyster Mushrooms:** The most delicate of the three with a light, almost sweet flavor, perfect for salads or gentle sautéing.

Black Pearl Mushrooms

Description:
Black Pearl mushrooms are a hybrid variety combining the traits of oyster and shiitake mushrooms. They have a smooth, dark cap and a flavor that combines both earthiness and mild seafood - like notes.

Common Culinary Uses:
These mushrooms are excellent in stir-fried dishes, soups, and as a meat substitute in vegetarian dishes due to their hearty texture and flavorful profile.

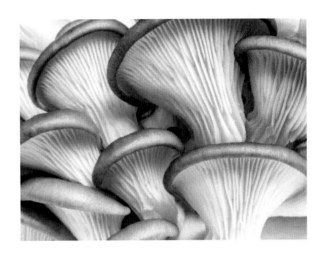

Maitake Mushrooms

Description:
Also known as Hen of the Woods, Maitake mushrooms grow in large clusters and have a rich, woodsy flavor. They are highly prized for their taste and potential health benefits.

Common Culinary Uses:
Maitake mushrooms are best used in dishes where their flavor can shine through, such as in sautés, grilled, or added to risottos. Their robust texture also makes them suitable for stews and soups where they can simmer and absorb flavors.

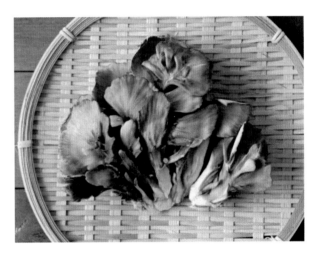

Health Benefits

Mushrooms are not only a delight for the palate but also offer numerous health and culinary benefits, making them a valuable addition to any diet. *(These statements have not been evaluated by the Food and Drug Administration.)*

Nutritional Value: Mushrooms are a low-calorie source of fiber, protein, and antioxidants. They also provide several important nutrients, including B vitamins (especially niacin, riboflavin, and pantothenic acid), selenium, potassium, copper, and even Vitamin D if they have been exposed to sunlight. This unique nutritional profile helps support vital bodily functions and contributes to overall health.

- **Immune Support:** Mushrooms are rich in beta-glucans, compounds that help boost the immune system. Certain mushroom varieties like shiitake, maitake, and reishi are particularly known for their immune-enhancing properties.

- **Cholesterol Management:** Some studies have shown that certain types of mushrooms can help lower cholesterol levels. The fibers and certain enzymes in mushrooms help to reduce cholesterol absorption and production in the liver.
- **Antioxidant Properties:** Mushrooms are a source of antioxidants like selenium, which help to combat free radicals in the body. This can reduce inflammation and protect against various chronic diseases.
- **Weight Management:** Due to their low calorie but high nutrient density, mushrooms are excellent for weight management diets. Their fibrous nature also helps in promoting satiety.
- **Blood Sugar Control:** The natural enzymes in mushrooms can also help to break down sugars and starches in the diet, which helps in controlling blood sugar levels.

Culinary Benefits:

- **Flavor Enhancement:** Mushrooms have a natural umami quality, which can enhance the flavor profile of any dish without the need for additional salt or fat. This makes them ideal for healthier cooking while maintaining robust flavors.
- **Texture Addition:** The variety of textures in mushrooms from chewy to tender allows them to be used in a multitude of culinary applications. They can be used as meat substitutes in vegetarian and vegan dishes, providing a satisfying texture.
- **Versatility in Recipes:** Mushrooms can be adapted to nearly any cooking method, including grilling, baking, frying, and stewing, and can be included in dishes ranging from appetizers and salads to main courses and even some desserts.

Incorporating mushrooms into your meals not only boosts nutritional intake and offers health benefits but also introduces new textures and flavors to your cooking, elevating everyday dishes into something special.

How to Store, Freeze, and Dry Mushrooms

Mushrooms are a versatile and nutritious ingredient but require proper handling to maintain their best quality. Here's how to store, freeze, and dry mushrooms effectively:

Guidelines for Proper Storage:

Refrigeration: Fresh mushrooms should be stored in the refrigerator. To maximize freshness, keep them in their original packaging or in a paper bag. Avoid plastic bags, as these can trap moisture and cause the mushrooms to spoil more quickly.

Avoid Washing: Do not wash mushrooms before storing them; moisture can hasten spoilage. Instead, brush off any dirt gently with a paper towel or soft brush and wash them just before use.

Ventilation: Ensure that there is adequate ventilation if not using original packaging. A partially opened bag or a container with a loose-fitting lid works well to allow some air circulation without drying out the mushrooms.

Instructions on How to Freeze Mushrooms:

Clean and Prepare: Wash the mushrooms and pat them dry. You can slice them if desired or leave them whole.

Blanch or Sauté: To maintain the best texture and flavor, it's advisable to blanch or sauté mushrooms before freezing. For blanching, boil them for 1-2 minutes, then plunge into ice water. For sautéing, cook in a small amount of butter or oil until slightly soft.

Cool Down: Ensure that the mushrooms are completely cool before freezing.

Pack and Freeze: Spread the cooled mushrooms on a baking sheet in a single layer. Freeze them until solid, then transfer to airtight containers or freezer bags. This prevents them from sticking together and allows you to use only the amount you need later.

Techniques for Drying Mushrooms:

Oven Drying: Place sliced mushrooms on a baking sheet in a single layer. Set the oven to the lowest temperature (150°F or 65°C, or the warm setting), and leave the door slightly ajar to allow moisture to escape. Dry them for 1-3 hours, checking frequently as cooking times can vary based on the oven and thickness of the slices.

Air Drying: In dry, warm climates, mushrooms can also be air-dried. String them on a thread and hang them in a dry, well-ventilated area away from direct sunlight. This process can take several days.

Dehydrator: If you have a dehydrator, follow the manufacturer's instructions for drying mushrooms. This method is more controlled and can yield more consistent results.

How to Rehydrate Dried Mushrooms:

Soaking: Place the dried mushrooms in a bowl and cover them with warm water. Let them soak for 20-30 minutes, or until they are fully rehydrated. The water used to rehydrate mushrooms is full of flavor and can be strained and used as a broth in cooking.

By following these guidelines, you can extend the shelf life of mushrooms, preserving their texture and flavor for use in many delicious recipes. Whether you choose to refrigerate, freeze, or dry your mushrooms, each method can help you enjoy this versatile ingredient throughout the season

Growing Mushrooms at Home

Growing mushrooms at home can be a rewarding hobby, offering fresh produce right from your kitchen or garden. You can find growing kits that make it really easy, or you can go all out and get a grow tent or mono-tub to grow them from a culture in a growing material.

Here are two easy ways to get started with home mushroom cultivation: from online mushroom grow supply companies:

Buy a complete home cultivation kit: Home mushroom cultivation kits are an excellent way for beginners to start growing mushrooms. These kits typically come with everything needed, including the spawn (mushroom strain), a growing medium infused with mushroom mycelium, and detailed instructions. Popular types of mushrooms to grow with kits include oyster, shiitake, and white button mushrooms. Kits simplify the process by controlling many variables that can affect mushroom growth, making them a user-friendly option.

Order the supplies separately and do it yourself: You can order a syringe of the mushroom strain (mycelium) and inject it into a sterilized bag of spawn (grain). Once the mycelium grows through the spawn grain bag contents, add it to a substrate (straw, woodchips, cardboard, coffee grounds or a manure/straw combo depending on the type of mushroom strain you are trying to grow.) You can order the mushroom strain, the pre-sterilized spawn and substrate directly from the online mushroom grow supplier.

Sterilization and preventing contamination is key, along with managing the temperature and humidity correctly.

It is so fun and rewarding to see your first mushrooms "fruit" and to use them in your cooking!

Check out the book "Growing Mushrooms at Home" by Ross Johnson for more details.

EASY MUSHROOM RECIPES

SIMPLE SAUTÉED BUTTON MUSHROOMS

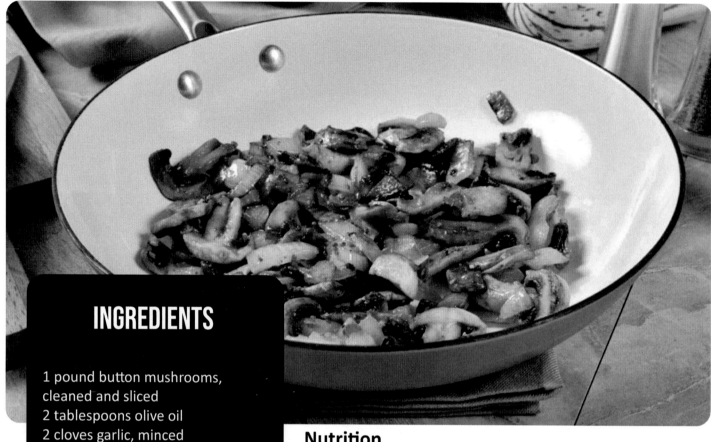

INGREDIENTS

1 pound button mushrooms, cleaned and sliced
2 tablespoons olive oil
2 cloves garlic, minced
1 tablespoon fresh thyme, chopped
Salt and crushed pepper to taste

Nutrition

Calories: 90, Protein: 3g, Carbohydrate: 4g, Fat: 7g

INSTRUCTIONS

1. Heat two tbsp oil in a skillet over medium heat.
2. Add mashed garlic to the skillet and sauté for about 1 minute until fragrant.
3. Increase the heat to medium-high and add the sliced mushrooms to the skillet. Cook for 8-10 minutes, stirring occasionally.
4. Sprinkle the chopped thyme over the mushrooms and powder it with salt and crushed pepper. Stir well to combine.
5. Serve immediately, adjusting seasoning if necessary.

 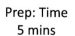

Prep: Time
5 mins

Cook Time
10 mins

Serving
4

MUSHROOM BRUSCHETTA

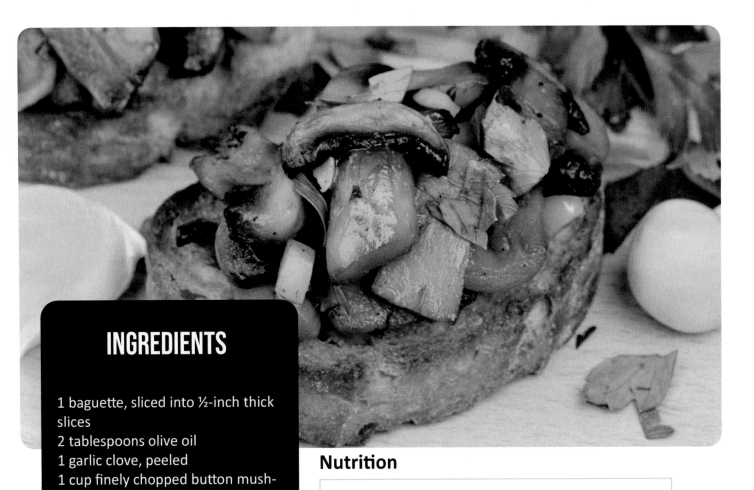

INGREDIENTS

1 baguette, sliced into ½-inch thick slices
2 tablespoons olive oil
1 garlic clove, peeled
1 cup finely chopped button mushrooms
1 tablespoon balsamic vinegar
2 tablespoons chopped fresh basil
Salt and crushed pepper to taste

Nutrition

Calories: 180, Protein: 6g, Carbohydrate: 25g, Fat: 7g

INSTRUCTIONS

1. Preheat oven to 400°F (200°C). Arrange the baguette slices on the paper-arranged baking sheet and brush every slice lightly with olive oil.
2. Bake in the oven for 5 minutes or until the edges are crisp and golden.
3. Massage the garlic clove over the toasted bread for a subtle garlic flavor.
4. In a skillet, heat the leftover oil over medium heat. Add the chopped mushrooms and sauté until they are soft and browned, about 5 minutes.
5. Remove and stir in the balsamic vinegar and basil. Powder it with salt and crushed pepper.
6. Spoon the mushroom mixture onto the toasted bread slices and serve immediately.

Prep: Time
10 mins

Cook Time
5 mins

Serving
4

MUSHROOM OMELET

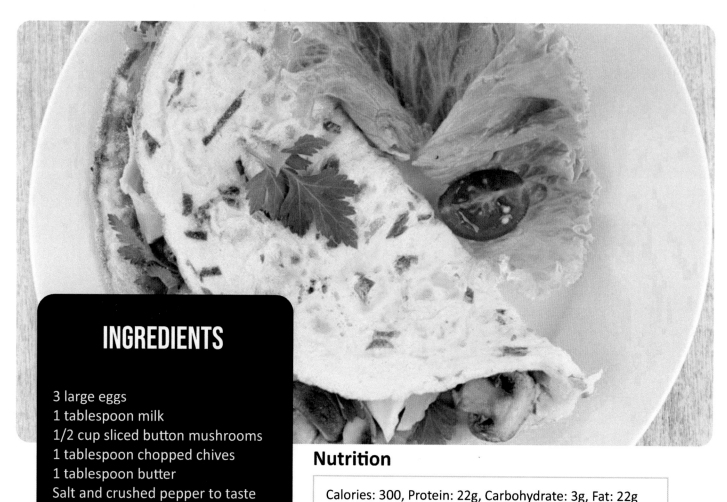

INGREDIENTS

3 large eggs
1 tablespoon milk
1/2 cup sliced button mushrooms
1 tablespoon chopped chives
1 tablespoon butter
Salt and crushed pepper to taste
1/4 cup shredded cheddar cheese
(optional)

Nutrition

Calories: 300, Protein: 22g, Carbohydrate: 3g, Fat: 22g

INSTRUCTIONS

1. In a mixing bowl, toss the eggs, milk, salt, and pepper.
2. Heat butter over medium heat. Add the mushrooms and sauté until tender and lightly browned about 5 minutes.
3. Ladle egg mixture over the mushrooms in the skillet, tilting the pan to spread evenly.
4. Sprinkle chives and cheese (if using) over the top. Cook for about 4-5 minutes, or until the eggs are set but still slightly runny on top.
5. Use a spatula to fold the omelet in half and slide onto a plate. Serve hot.

Prep: Time
5 mins

Cook Time
10 mins

Serving
1

GARLIC MUSHROOM PASTA

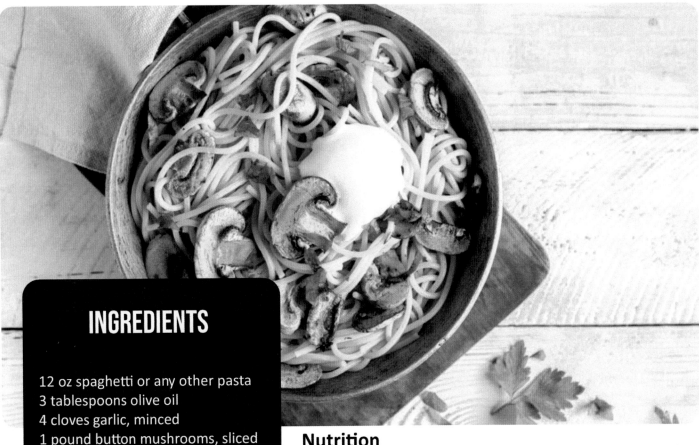

INGREDIENTS

12 oz spaghetti or any other pasta
3 tablespoons olive oil
4 cloves garlic, minced
1 pound button mushrooms, sliced
1/4 cup white wine (optional)
1/4 cup fresh parsley, chopped
Salt and crushed pepper to taste
Grated Parmesan cheese for serving

Nutrition

Calories: 420, Protein: 14g, Carbohydrate: 65g, Fat: 12g

INSTRUCTIONS

1. Prepare pasta according to the steps mentioned on the package until al dente. Drain and set aside, reserving 1 cup of pasta water.
2. Heat one tbsp oil in a skillet over medium heat. Add garlic and sauté for 1 minute until fragrant.
3. Add mushroom slices and cook for 8 minutes.
4. If using, pour in the white wine and let it reduce for about 2 minutes.
5. Toss the prepared pasta with the mushroom mixture, adding reserved water to create a light sauce.
6. Stir in the chopped parsley, powder it with salt and crushed pepper, and serve topped with grated Parmesan cheese.

Prep: Time
10 mins

Cook Time
15 mins

Serving
4

MUSHROOM AND BELL PEPPER STIR-FRY

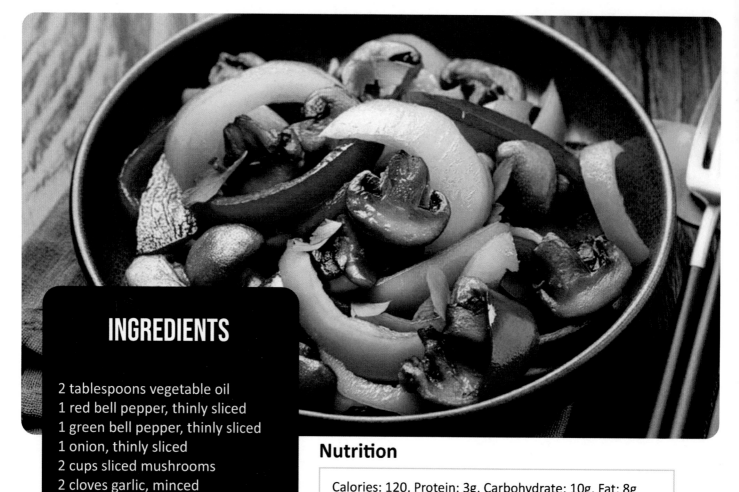

INGREDIENTS

2 tablespoons vegetable oil
1 red bell pepper, thinly sliced
1 green bell pepper, thinly sliced
1 onion, thinly sliced
2 cups sliced mushrooms
2 cloves garlic, minced
2 tablespoons soy sauce
1 tablespoon oyster sauce
1 teaspoon sesame oil

Nutrition

Calories: 120, Protein: 3g, Carbohydrate: 10g, Fat: 8g

INSTRUCTIONS

1. Heat two tbsp vegetable oil in a skillet/wok over high heat.
2. Add the bell peppers and onion, stir-frying for about 3 minutes until just tender.
3. Add the mushrooms and garlic, continuing to stir-fry for another 5 minutes until the mushrooms are cooked and the vegetables are crisp-tender.
4. Stir in soy sauce, oyster sauce, and sesame oil, mixing well.
5. Serve immediately, ideally over steamed rice or noodles.

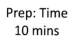

Prep: Time
10 mins

Cook Time
10 mins

Serving
4

BAKED MUSHROOM AND CHEESE FRITTATA

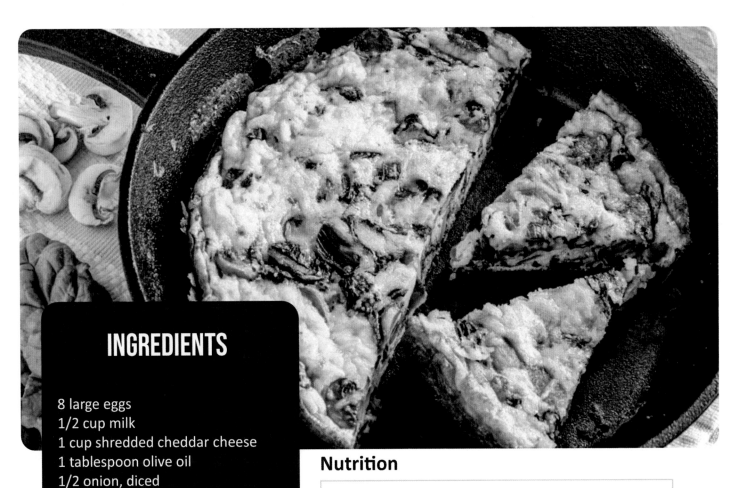

INGREDIENTS

8 large eggs
1/2 cup milk
1 cup shredded cheddar cheese
1 tablespoon olive oil
1/2 onion, diced
1 cup sliced mushrooms
Salt and crushed pepper to taste
Fresh herbs (any parsley or chives)
for garnish
1 cup of fresh spinach (optional)

Nutrition

Calories: 230, Protein: 16g, Carbohydrate: 5g, Fat: 17g

INSTRUCTIONS

1. Instructions:
2. Preheat oven to 375°F (190°C).
3. In a bowl, pulse the eggs, milk, salt, and pepper. Stir in the cheese. (and spinach if you choose)
4. Heat one tbsp oil in an oven-safe skillet over medium heat. Sauté onion until translucent, about 5 minutes.
5. Add mushroom slices and cook until they are soft and browned, about 5 more minutes.
6. Ladle egg mixture over the mushrooms and onions. Cook without stirring for 2 minutes to allow the edges to set.
7. Put the skillet and bake for 18-20 minutes or until the frittata is set and lightly golden on top.
8. Garnish with fresh herbs before serving.

Prep: Time   Cook Time   Serving
10 mins   25 mins   6

MUSHROOM RISOTTO

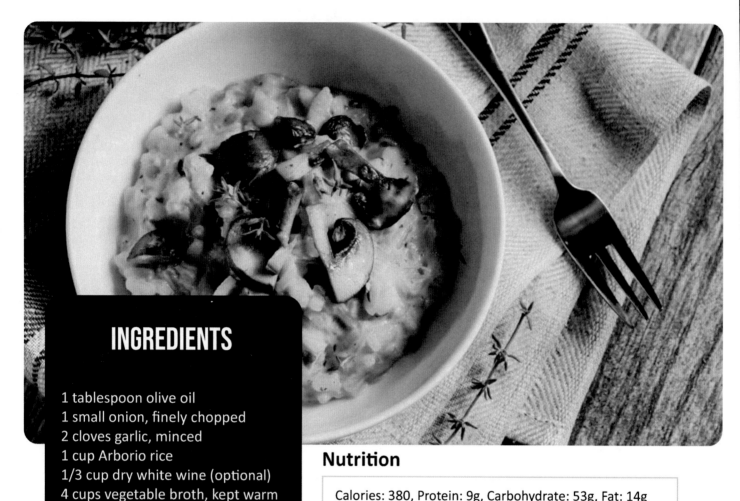

INGREDIENTS

1 tablespoon olive oil
1 small onion, finely chopped
2 cloves garlic, minced
1 cup Arborio rice
1/3 cup dry white wine (optional)
4 cups vegetable broth, kept warm
1 cup sliced button mushrooms
1 cup sliced cremini mushrooms
1/4 cup grated Parmesan cheese
2 tablespoons unsalted butter
Salt and crushed pepper to taste
Fresh parsley, chopped (for garnish)

Nutrition

Calories: 380, Protein: 9g, Carbohydrate: 53g, Fat: 14g

INSTRUCTIONS

1. Heat one tbsp oil in a large saucepan over medium heat. Add onion and mashed garlic, sauté until the onion is translucent, for about 5 minutes.
2. Add the Arborio rice, stirring to coat with oil for about 2 minutes.
3. Ladle white wine (if you have) and cook until it has mostly evaporated.
4. Add one cup of warm vegetable broth to the rice, stirring continuously until the broth is absorbed. Repeat this process with the leftover broth for 18-20 minutes total.
5. In a separate skillet, sauté the mushrooms in butter until they are golden and soft.
6. Fold the cooked mushrooms, Parmesan cheese, and additional butter into the risotto. Powder it with salt and crushed pepper to taste.
7. Serve with chopped parsley and additional Parmesan if desired.

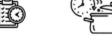

Prep: Time
10 mins

Cook Time
25 mins

Serving
4

21

MUSHROOM GRAVY

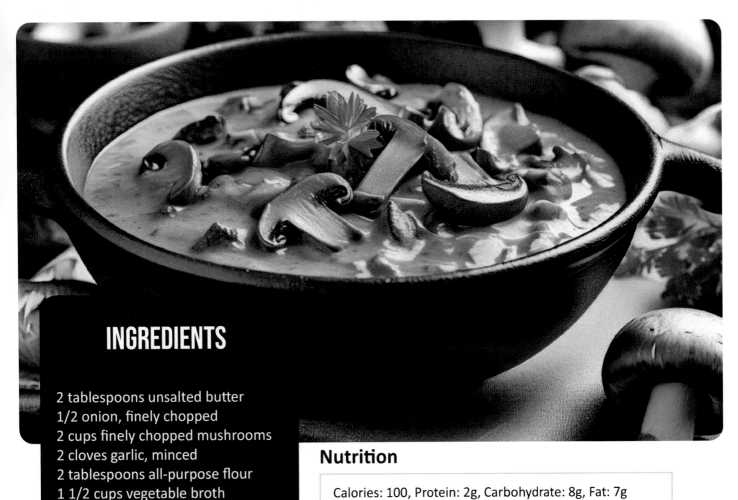

INGREDIENTS

2 tablespoons unsalted butter
1/2 onion, finely chopped
2 cups finely chopped mushrooms
2 cloves garlic, minced
2 tablespoons all-purpose flour
1 1/2 cups vegetable broth
1 teaspoon soy sauce
Salt and crushed pepper to taste
Fresh thyme, chopped (optional, for garnish)

Nutrition

Calories: 100, Protein: 2g, Carbohydrate: 8g, Fat: 7g

INSTRUCTIONS

1. Melt the butter pan over medium heat. Add onion and mashed garlic, and cook until the onion is translucent, for about 5 minutes.
2. Add the chopped mushrooms, cooking until they are soft and browned, about 5 more minutes.
3. Sprinkle flour, stirring to coat them, and cook for one minute.
4. Gradually whisk in the vegetable broth and soy sauce, ensuring no lumps form.
5. Bring to a simmer, and keep stirring until the gravy thickens about 5 minutes.
6. Powder it with salt and crushed pepper to taste. Serve hot, garnished with chopped thyme if using.

Prep: Time
5 mins

Cook Time
15 mins

Serving
4

BREAKFAST

MUSHROOM SPINACH BREAKFAST SKILLET

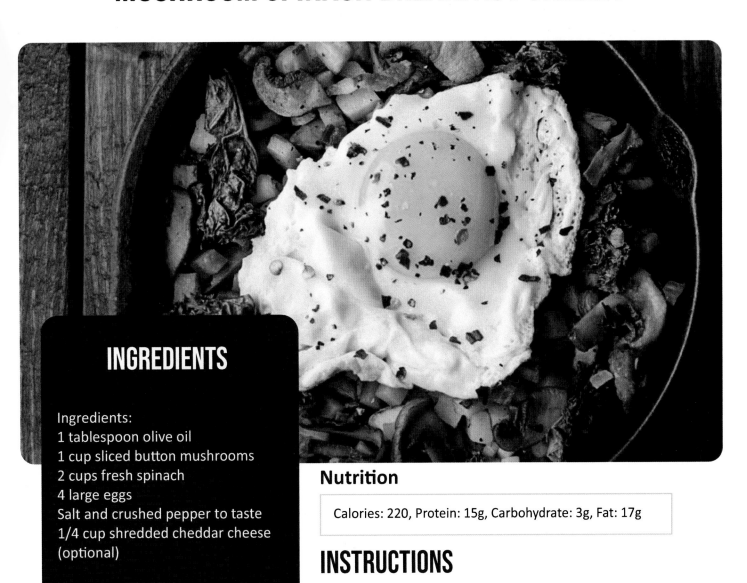

INGREDIENTS

Ingredients:
1 tablespoon olive oil
1 cup sliced button mushrooms
2 cups fresh spinach
4 large eggs
Salt and crushed pepper to taste
1/4 cup shredded cheddar cheese
(optional)

Nutrition

Calories: 220, Protein: 15g, Carbohydrate: 3g, Fat: 17g

INSTRUCTIONS

1. Heat one tbsp oil in a skillet over medium heat. Add mushroom slices and sauté until they are golden and tender, about 5 minutes.
2. Add spinach and cook to wilted, about 2 minutes. Make four wells and crack one egg into each well.
3. Powder it with salt and crushed pepper. Cover with its lid and cook until the egg whites, about 3-4 minutes.
4. Sprinkle with shredded cheddar cheese, if using, and serve directly from the skillet.

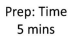

Prep: Time
5 mins

Cook Time
10 mins

Serving
2

CHEESY MUSHROOM BREAKFAST TACOS

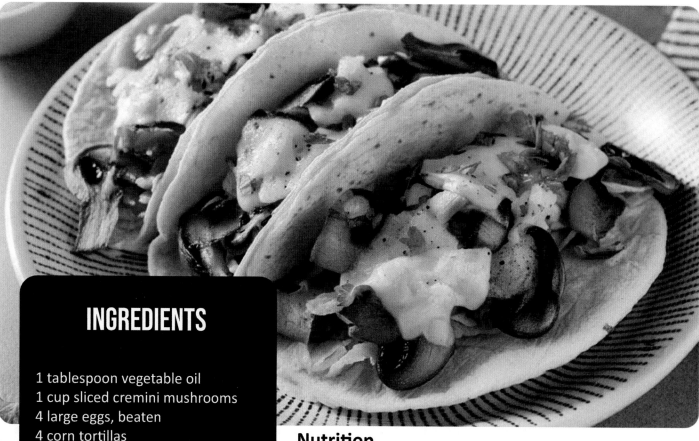

INGREDIENTS

1 tablespoon vegetable oil
1 cup sliced cremini mushrooms
4 large eggs, beaten
4 corn tortillas
1/2 cup shredded Monterey Jack cheese
Salt and crushed pepper to taste
Fresh cilantro, chopped (for garnish)
Salsa, for serving

Nutrition

Calories: 180, Protein: 10g, Carbohydrate: 14g, Fat: 10g

INSTRUCTIONS

1. Heat one tbsp oil in a skillet over medium heat. Add sliced cremini mushrooms and cook for 5 minutes.
2. Pour the beaten eggs over the mushrooms, stirring gently to scramble with the mushrooms until the eggs are cooked through.
3. Warm the tortillas. Spoon the mushroom and egg mixture into each tortilla. Top with shredded cheese, cilantro, and a spoonful of salsa.
4. Fold the tortillas over and serve immediately.

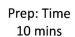

Prep: Time
10 mins

Cook Time
5 mins

Serving
4

MUSHROOM AND FETA BREAKFAST BURRITOS

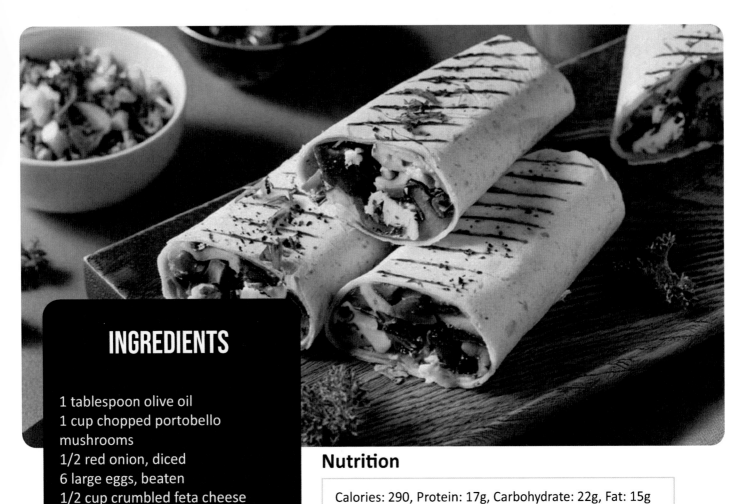

INGREDIENTS

1 tablespoon olive oil
1 cup chopped portobello mushrooms
1/2 red onion, diced
6 large eggs, beaten
1/2 cup crumbled feta cheese
4 flour tortillas
Salt and crushed pepper to taste
Fresh spinach leaves (optional)

Nutrition

Calories: 290, Protein: 17g, Carbohydrate: 22g, Fat: 15g

INSTRUCTIONS

1. Heat one tbsp oil in a skillet over medium heat. Add the mushrooms and onion, sauté until the mushrooms and onion for 5 minutes.
2. Drop the pulsed eggs over the mushroom onion and onion mixture, stirring to scramble the eggs as they cook.
3. Remove and toss in crumbled feta cheese. Powder it with salt and crushed pepper.
4. Warm the tortillas. Divide the egg mixture among the tortillas, adding fresh spinach if desired. Roll up the tortillas to form burritos.
5. Serve immediately.

 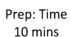

Prep: Time
10 mins

Cook Time
10 mins

Serving
4

SAVORY MUSHROOM AND HERB PANCAKES

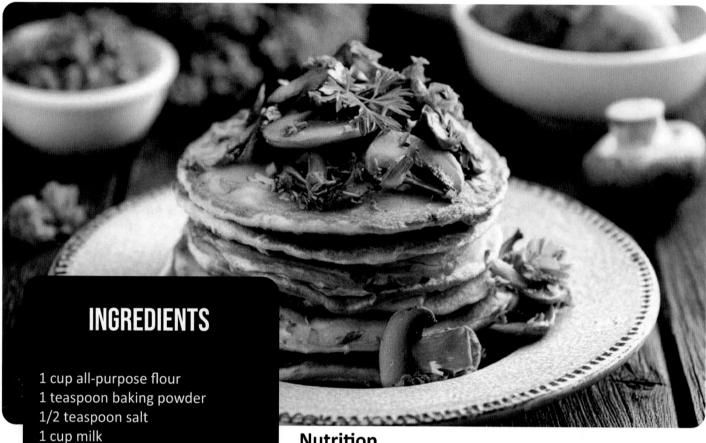

INGREDIENTS

1 cup all-purpose flour
1 teaspoon baking powder
1/2 teaspoon salt
1 cup milk
1 egg
2 tablespoons melted butter
1 cup finely chopped mushrooms
1/4 cup chopped herbs (parsley, chives, and thyme)
Additional butter or oil for cooking

Nutrition

Calories: 260, Protein: 9g, Carbohydrate: 29g, Fat: 12g

INSTRUCTIONS

1. Take the large shallow bowl and toss the flour, baking powder, and salt.
2. Take the other shallow bowl and beat together the milk, egg, and melted butter.
3. Toss the milk mixture into the flour mixture until just combined.
4. Fold in the chopped mushrooms and herbs.
5. Put the non-stick skillet over moderate heat and brush with butter or oil. Drop 1/4 cup batter for one pancake and cook until bubble appears on the upper surface, then flip and cook for 2-3 minutes more.
6. Serve warm with sour cream or your choice of toppings.

Prep: Time
15 mins

Cook Time
20 mins

Serving
4

MUSHROOM AND GRUYERE QUICHE

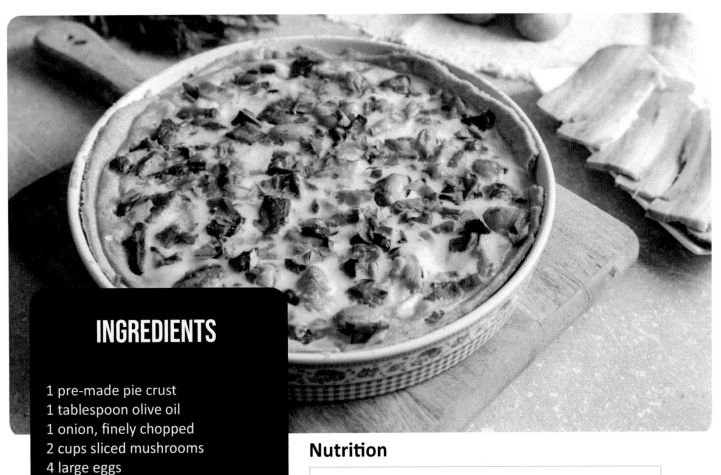

INGREDIENTS

1 pre-made pie crust
1 tablespoon olive oil
1 onion, finely chopped
2 cups sliced mushrooms
4 large eggs
1 cup cream
1 cup grated Gruyere cheese
Salt and crushed pepper to taste
Fresh thyme leaves for garnish

Nutrition

Calories: 410, Protein: 16g, Carbohydrate: 18g, Fat: 31g

INSTRUCTIONS

1. Preheat oven to 375°F (190°C). Put the pie crust in a 9-inch pie dish.
2. Heat one tbsp oil in a skillet over medium heat. Add onion and mushrooms, and cook until both are soft and golden, for about 10 minutes.
3. Take the large shallow bowl and toss the eggs and cream. Stir in the cooked mushrooms and onions and Gruyere cheese, and powder it with salt and crushed pepper.
4. Ladle the mixture into the prepared pie crust.
5. Bake for 25 minutes until the quiche is set and the top is lightly browned.
6. Garnish with thyme leaves before serving.

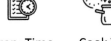

Prep: Time
15 mins

Cook Time
35 mins

Serving
6

MUSHROOM AND CHEDDAR BREAKFAST STRATA

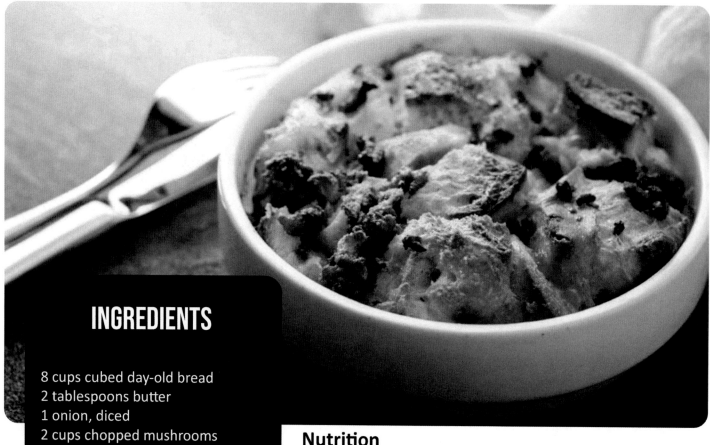

INGREDIENTS

8 cups cubed day-old bread
2 tablespoons butter
1 onion, diced
2 cups chopped mushrooms
8 large eggs
2 cups milk
1 teaspoon mustard powder
2 cups shredded cheddar cheese
Salt and crushed pepper to taste
Fresh parsley, chopped (for garnish)

Nutrition

Calories: 350, Protein: 20g, Carbohydrate: 24g, Fat: 20g

INSTRUCTIONS

1. Grease the 9x13-inch rectangular baking dish and spread the bread cubes evenly in the dish.
2. Melt butter over medium heat. Add chopped onion and mushrooms, and cook for 10 minutes.
3. Scatter the mushroom mixture over the bread.
4. Take the large shallow bowl and toss the eggs, milk, mustard powder, salt, and pepper. Stir in the cheddar cheese.
5. Ladle the egg mixture over the bread and mushrooms. Cover and refrigerate overnight.
6. Preheat oven to 350°F (175°C). Bake the strata for 45 minutes or until puffed and golden.
7. Garnish with chopped parsley before serving.

 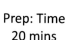

Prep: Time   Cook Time   Serving
20 mins   45 mins   8

MUSHROOM AND ZUCCHINI BREAKFAST HASH

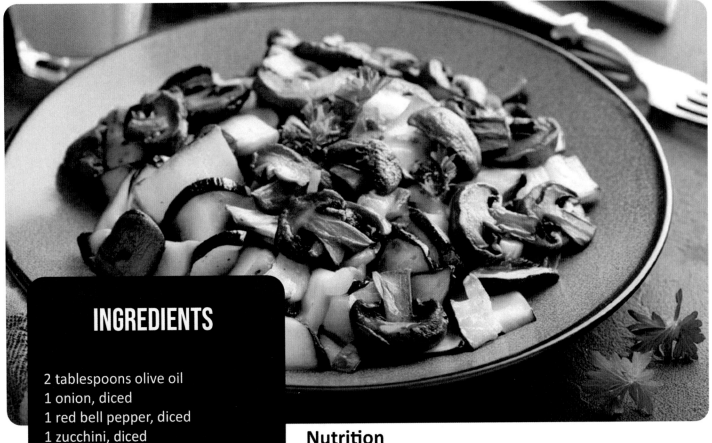

INGREDIENTS

2 tablespoons olive oil
1 onion, diced
1 red bell pepper, diced
1 zucchini, diced
2 cups chopped mushrooms (such as button or cremini)
Salt and crushed pepper to taste
4 large eggs
Fresh parsley, chopped (for garnish)

Nutrition

Calories: 220, Protein: 12g, Carbohydrate: 10g, Fat: 15g

INSTRUCTIONS

1. Heat one tbsp oil in a skillet over medium heat. Add diced onion, diced bell pepper, cooking until they begin to soften, about 5 minutes.
2. Add the zucchini and mushrooms to the skillet, seasoning with salt and pepper. Cook, stirring occasionally, until the veggies get tender and lightly browned, about 10 minutes.
3. Make four wells and crack eggs into every well. Cover it with its lid and cook for 4-5 minutes for runny yolks.
4. Garnish with chopped parsley and serve immediately.

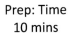
Prep: Time
10 mins

Cook Time
15 mins

Serving
4

CREAMY MUSHROOM AND LEEK BAKED EGGS

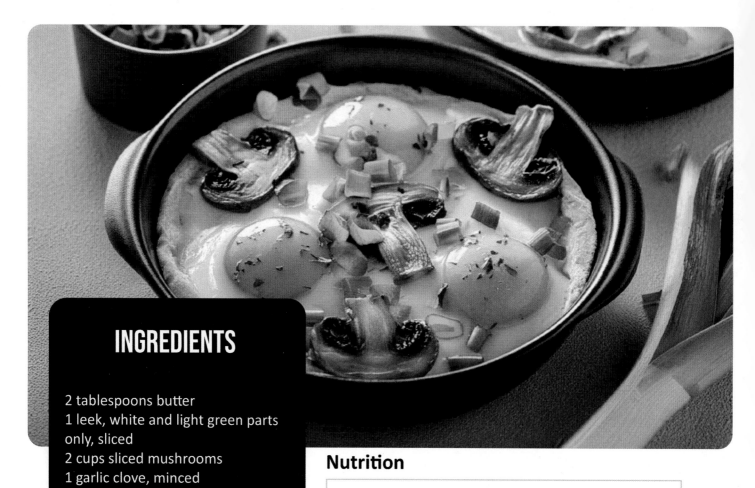

INGREDIENTS

2 tablespoons butter
1 leek, white and light green parts only, sliced
2 cups sliced mushrooms
1 garlic clove, minced
1/2 cup heavy cream
Salt and crushed pepper to taste
4 large eggs
2 tablespoons grated Parmesan cheese
Fresh chives, chopped (for garnish)

Nutrition

Calories: 290, Protein: 10g, Carbohydrate: 6g, Fat: 25g

INSTRUCTIONS

1. Preheat oven to 375°F (190°C).
2. Melt butter over medium heat. Add chopped leek and mushrooms, cooking until they are soft and the moisture has evaporated, about 10 minutes. Add garlic and cook for another minute.
3. Add heavy cream, stir well, and simmer until slightly thickened, about 3 minutes. Powder it with salt and crushed pepper.
4. Divide the mushroom and leek mixture among four small baking dishes. Crack an egg into each dish and sprinkle with Parmesan cheese.
5. Bake for 7-10 minutes.
6. Garnish with chopped chives and serve hot.

Prep: Time
10 mins

Cook Time
20 mins

Serving
4

SAUCES & SOUPS

CLASSIC CREAM OF MUSHROOM SOUP

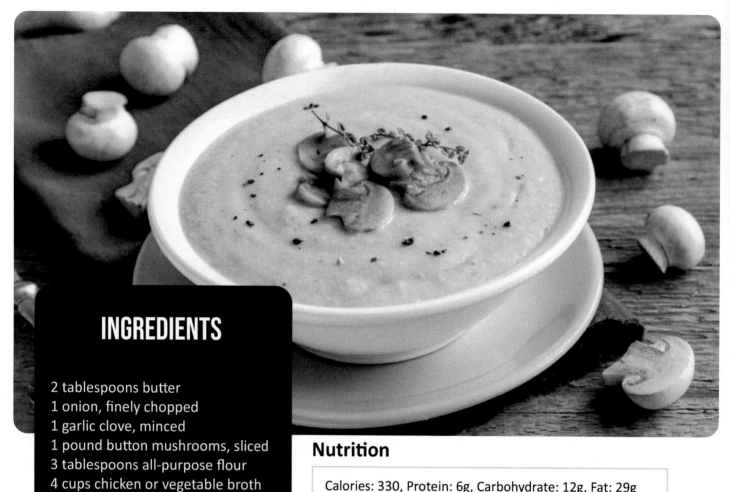

INGREDIENTS

2 tablespoons butter
1 onion, finely chopped
1 garlic clove, minced
1 pound button mushrooms, sliced
3 tablespoons all-purpose flour
4 cups chicken or vegetable broth
1 cup heavy cream
Salt and crushed pepper to taste
Fresh parsley, chopped (for garnish)

Nutrition

Calories: 330, Protein: 6g, Carbohydrate: 12g, Fat: 29g

INSTRUCTIONS

1. Melt butter in a saucepan over moderate flame. Add diced onion and garlic, cooking until softened, about 5 minutes.
2. Add mushroom slices and cook until they have released their juices and are golden brown, about 10 minutes.
3. Sprinkle flour and stir to combine. Cook for 2 minutes to discard the raw taste.
4. Gradually add the broth, stirring constantly to prevent lumps. Take it to a simmer and cook for 10 minutes.
5. Puree the soup in the food blender until smooth (or in batches using a regular blender).
6. Stir in the cream and heat through. Powder it with salt and crushed pepper to taste.
7. Serve garnished with chopped parsley.

Prep: Time	Cook Time	Serving
10 mins	20 mins	4

PORCINI MUSHROOM AND ROSEMARY SAUCE

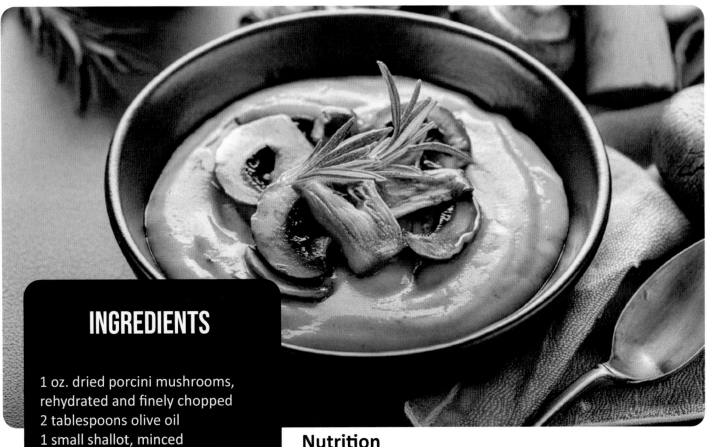

INGREDIENTS

1 oz. dried porcini mushrooms, rehydrated and finely chopped
2 tablespoons olive oil
1 small shallot, minced
2 cloves garlic, minced
1 tablespoon fresh rosemary, finely chopped
1 cup beef or vegetable broth
1/2 cup heavy cream
Salt and crushed pepper to taste

Nutrition

Calories: 180, Protein: 2g, Carbohydrate: 4g, Fat: 17g

INSTRUCTIONS

1. Heat one tbsp oil in a saucepan over medium heat. Add shallot and garlic, cooking until translucent, about 3 minutes.
2. Add the chopped porcini mushrooms and rosemary. Cook for another 5 minutes, until fragrant.
3. Ladle in the broth and bring to a simmer. Decrease the stove heat and simmer for 5 minutes.
4. Toss in cream and simmer until the sauce has thickened slightly about 5 minutes.
5. Powder it with salt and crushed pepper to taste. Serve over pasta, steaks, or roasted vegetables.

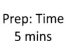
Prep: Time
5 mins

Cook Time
15 mins

Serving
4

SHIITAKE MUSHROOM MISO SOUP

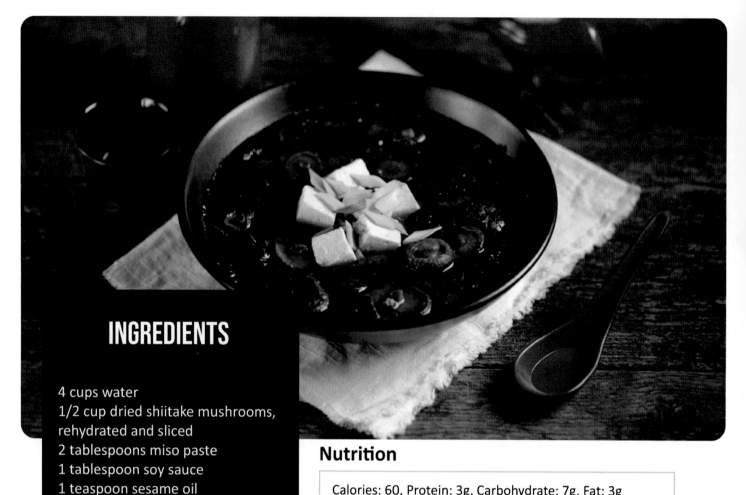

INGREDIENTS

4 cups water
1/2 cup dried shiitake mushrooms, rehydrated and sliced
2 tablespoons miso paste
1 tablespoon soy sauce
1 teaspoon sesame oil
2 green onions, chopped
Tofu cubes (optional)

Nutrition

Calories: 60, Protein: 3g, Carbohydrate: 7g, Fat: 3g

INSTRUCTIONS

1. Add water to a simmer in a moderate pot. Add sliced shiitake mushrooms and cook for about 5 minutes.
2. In a small, deep-bottom bowl, mix the miso paste with water (hot) until smooth, then stir back into the pot.
3. Add soy sauce and sesame oil to the soup and stir to combine.
4. Add green onions and tofu cubes, if using, and simmer for another 5 minutes.
5. Serve hot, avoiding boiling the soup after adding the miso to preserve its flavors and health benefits.

Prep: Time
10 mins

Cook Time
10 mins

Serving
4

CREAMY MUSHROOM AND LEEK SOUP

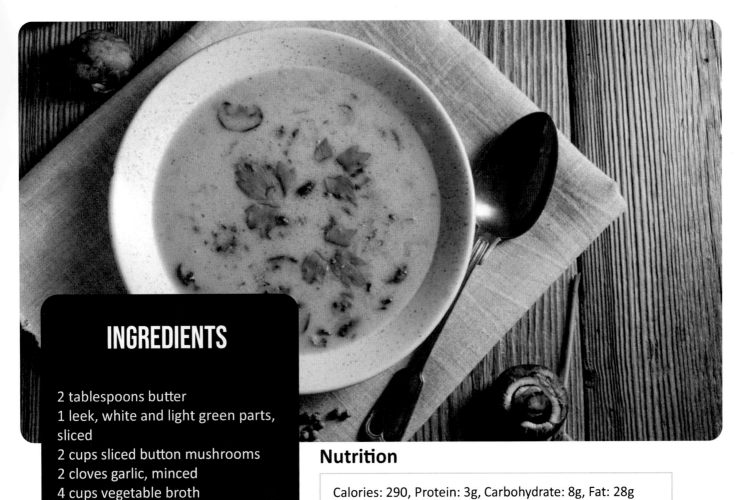

INGREDIENTS

2 tablespoons butter
1 leek, white and light green parts, sliced
2 cups sliced button mushrooms
2 cloves garlic, minced
4 cups vegetable broth
1 cup heavy cream
Salt and crushed pepper to taste
Fresh chives, chopped (for garnish)

Nutrition

Calories: 290, Protein: 3g, Carbohydrate: 8g, Fat: 28g

INSTRUCTIONS

1. Melt butter in a deep-bottom pot over medium heat. Add the leek and garlic, sauté until the leek is soft, for about 5 minutes.
2. Add mushroom slices and cook until they are golden and softened about 10 minutes.
3. Ladle in vegetable broth and bring to a boil. Reduce heat and simmer for 10 minutes.
4. Blend the soup in the food blender until smooth. Toss
5. the heavy cream and heat through. Powder it with salt and crushed pepper to taste.
6. Serve hot, garnished with chopped chives.

 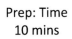

Prep: Time
10 mins

Cook Time
25 mins

Serving
4

SPICY MUSHROOM AND TOMATO SAUCE

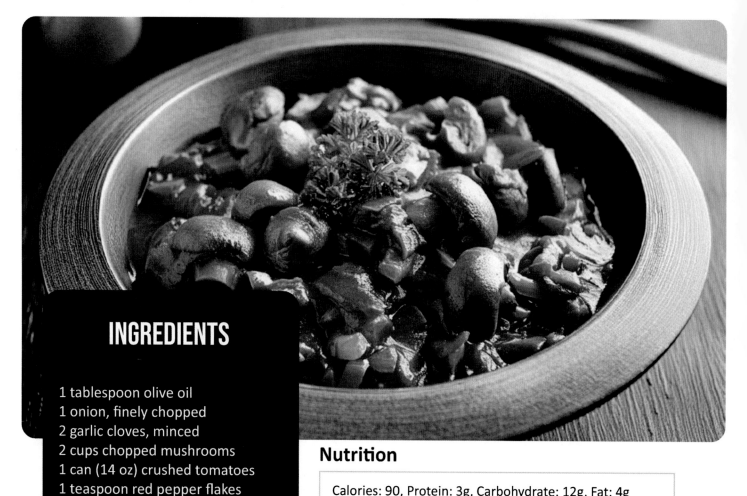

INGREDIENTS

1 tablespoon olive oil
1 onion, finely chopped
2 garlic cloves, minced
2 cups chopped mushrooms
1 can (14 oz) crushed tomatoes
1 teaspoon red pepper flakes
1 teaspoon dried oregano
Salt and crushed pepper, to taste
Fresh basil, torn (for garnish)

Nutrition

Calories: 90, Protein: 3g, Carbohydrate: 12g, Fat: 4g

INSTRUCTIONS

1. Heat one tbsp oil in a saucepan over medium heat. Add diced onion and mashed garlic, cooking until onion is translucent, about 5 minutes.
2. Add 2 cups chopped mushroom and cook for 5 minutes.
3. Stir in crushed tomatoes, red pepper flakes, and oregano. Simmer for 7-10 minutes, to meld the flavours.
4. Powder it with salt and crushed pepper. Serve over pasta or as a sauce for grilled meats, garnished with fresh basil.

Prep: Time   Cook Time   Serving
5 mins   20 mins   4

MUSHROOM AND ROASTED GARLIC ALFREDO SAUCE

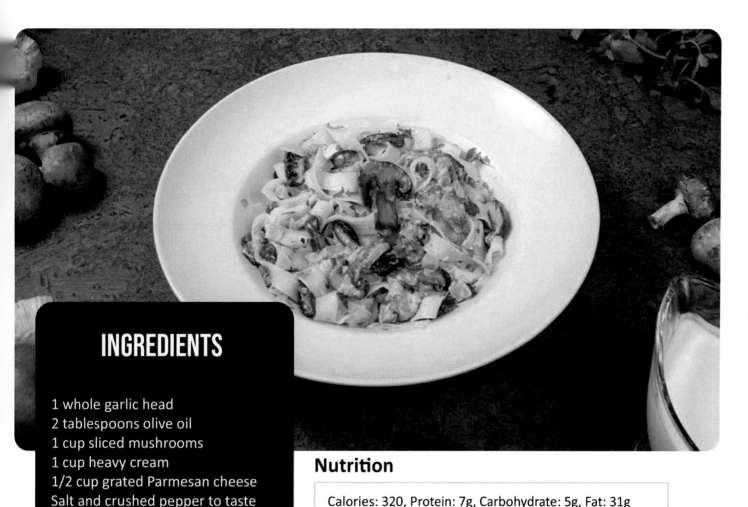

INGREDIENTS

1 whole garlic head
2 tablespoons olive oil
1 cup sliced mushrooms
1 cup heavy cream
1/2 cup grated Parmesan cheese
Salt and crushed pepper to taste
Fresh parsley, chopped (for garnish)

Nutrition

Calories: 320, Protein: 7g, Carbohydrate: 5g, Fat: 31g

INSTRUCTIONS

1. Preheat oven to 400°F (200°C). Slice the top off the head of garlic, drizzle with one tbsp oil, wrap in foil, and roast for 20 minutes.
2. Heat leftover oil over moderate heat. Add mushrooms and sauté until golden and tender, about 5 minutes.
3. Squeeze out the skins of the roasted garlic cloves and add them to the skillet with the mushrooms. Mash with a fork.
4. Add heavy cream and take it to a simmer. Stir in grated Parmesan until the sauce thickens, about 5 minutes.
5. Powder it with salt and crushed pepper. Serve over pasta, garnished with chopped parsley.

Prep: Time
15 mins

Cook Time
20 mins

Serving
4

GOLDEN OYSTER MUSHROOM BISQUE

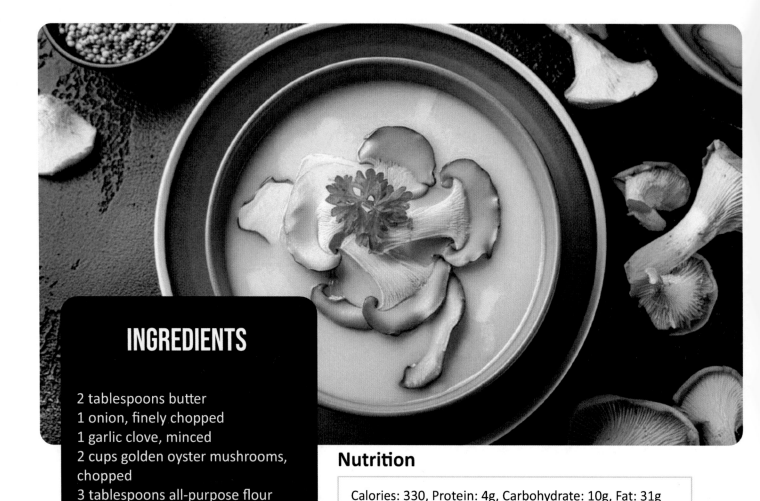

INGREDIENTS

2 tablespoons butter
1 onion, finely chopped
1 garlic clove, minced
2 cups golden oyster mushrooms, chopped
3 tablespoons all-purpose flour
4 cups chicken or vegetable broth
1 cup heavy cream
Salt and crushed pepper to taste
Fresh chives, chopped (for garnish)

Nutrition

Calories: 330, Protein: 4g, Carbohydrate: 10g, Fat: 31g

INSTRUCTIONS

1. Melt butter in a deep-bottom pot over medium heat. Add diced onion and mashed garlic, cooking until onion is translucent, about 5 minutes.
2. Add golden oyster mushrooms and cook until they are soft and have released their moisture, about 5 minutes.
3. Sprinkle flour and stir to coat. Cook for one minute to discard the raw flour taste.
4. Gradually add broth, stirring continuously, and bring to a simmer. Cook for 10 minutes.
5. Use the regular food blender to blend the soup until smooth.
6. Toss
7. in the heavy cream and heat thoroughly without boiling. Powder it with salt and crushed pepper to taste.
8. Serve hot, garnished with chopped chives.

Prep: Time	Cook Time	Serving
10 mins	20 mins	4

EARTHY MUSHROOM AND BARLEY SOUP

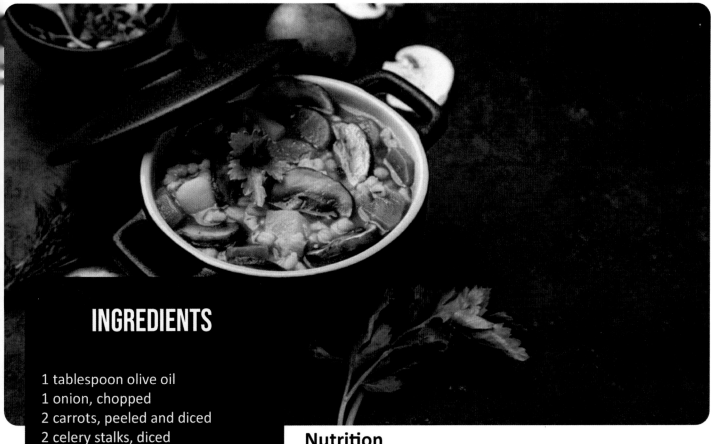

INGREDIENTS

1 tablespoon olive oil
1 onion, chopped
2 carrots, peeled and diced
2 celery stalks, diced
2 cups mixed mushrooms (such as button, cremini, and shiitake), chopped
1 cup pearl barley
6 cups vegetable broth
2 teaspoons fresh thyme leaves
Salt and crushed pepper to taste
Fresh parsley, chopped (for garnish)

Nutrition

Calories: 180, Protein: 4g, Carbohydrate: 32g, Fat: 4g

INSTRUCTIONS

1. Heat one tbsp oil in a deep-bottom pot over medium heat. Add chopped onion, carrots, and diced celery, and cook until the veggies get softened, for about 5 minutes.
2. Add mushroom slices and cook until they are browned and tender, about 10 minutes.
3. Stir in barley and vegetable broth. Bring to a boil, then decrease the stove heat to low and simmer, covered with a lid, until the barley is tender, about 25 minutes.
4. Add thyme and powder it with salt and crushed pepper. Simmer for an additional 5 minutes.
5. Serve hot, garnished with chopped parsley.

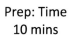

Prep: Time
10 mins

Cook Time
40 mins

Serving
6

APPETIZERS

MUSHROOM CAPRESE BITES

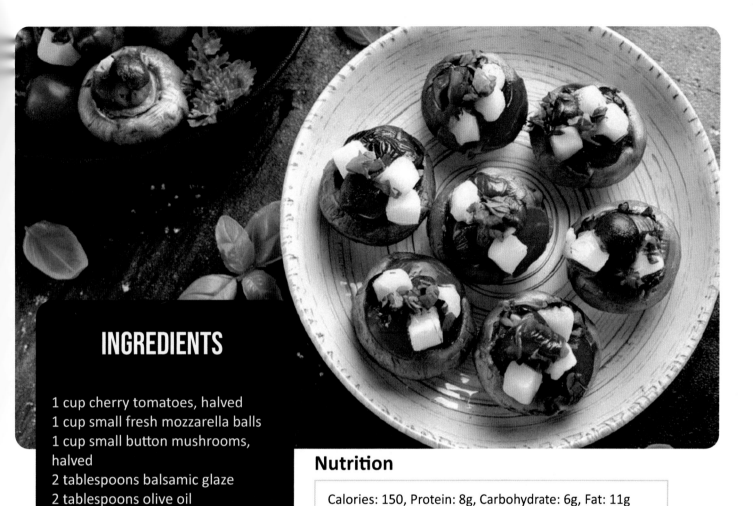

INGREDIENTS

1 cup cherry tomatoes, halved
1 cup small fresh mozzarella balls
1 cup small button mushrooms, halved
2 tablespoons balsamic glaze
2 tablespoons olive oil
Fresh basil leaves for garnish
Salt and crushed pepper to taste

Nutrition

Calories: 150, Protein: 8g, Carbohydrate: 6g, Fat: 11g

INSTRUCTIONS

1. In a mixing bowl, combine cherry tomatoes, mozzarella balls, and button mushrooms.
2. Drizzle with olive oil and balsamic glaze. Gently toss to coat evenly.
3. Powder it with salt and crushed pepper.
4. Arrange on skewers, alternating between tomato, mozzarella, and mushroom, with a basil leaf between each.
5. Serve immediately or refrigerate until serving.

Prep: Time
15 mins

Cook Time
00 mins

Serving
4

MUSHROOM-STUFFED MINI BELL PEPPERS

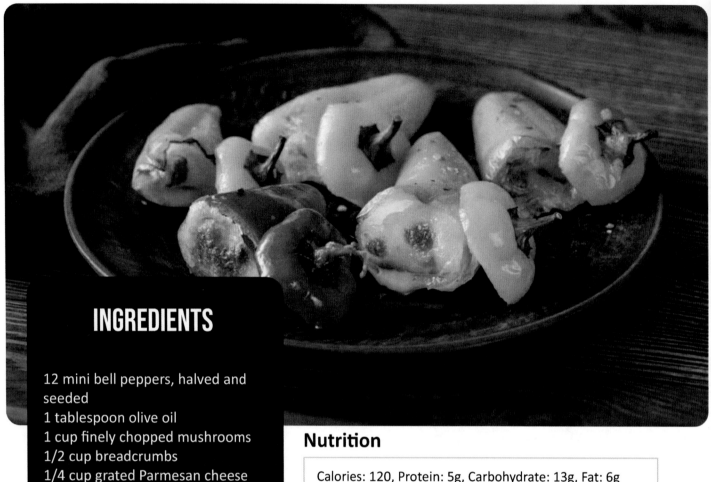

INGREDIENTS

12 mini bell peppers, halved and seeded
1 tablespoon olive oil
1 cup finely chopped mushrooms
1/2 cup breadcrumbs
1/4 cup grated Parmesan cheese
2 cloves garlic, minced
Salt and crushed pepper to taste
Fresh parsley, chopped (for garnish)

Nutrition

Calories: 120, Protein: 5g, Carbohydrate: 13g, Fat: 6g

INSTRUCTIONS

1. Preheat oven to 375°F (190°C).
2. Heat one tbsp oil in a skillet over medium heat. Add mushrooms and garlic, cooking until mushrooms are golden and moisture has evaporated about 5 minutes.
3. Remove from heat. Stir in breadcrumbs and Parmesan cheese. Powder it with salt and crushed pepper.
4. Stuff each bell pepper half with the mushroom mixture.
5. Arrange stuffed peppers on a baking sheet. Bake for 15 minutes.
6. Garnish with chopped parsley before serving.

Prep: Time
20 mins

Cook Time
15 mins

Serving
4

MUSHROOM AND CREAM CHEESE TARTLETS

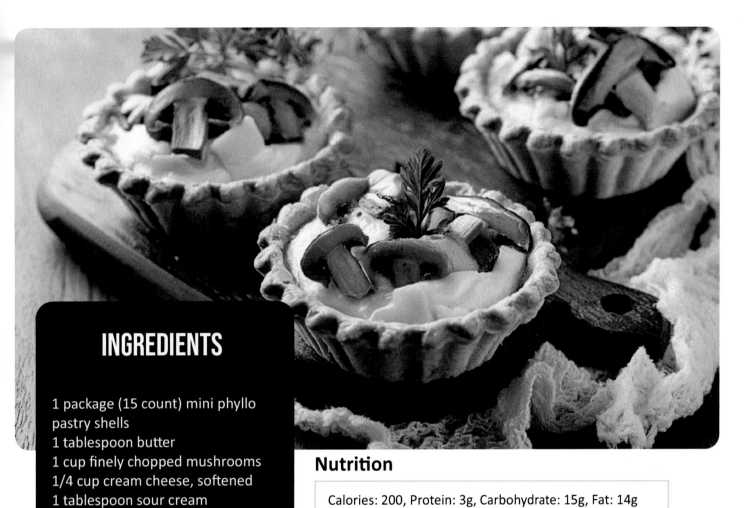

INGREDIENTS

1 package (15 count) mini phyllo pastry shells
1 tablespoon butter
1 cup finely chopped mushrooms
1/4 cup cream cheese, softened
1 tablespoon sour cream
1/4 teaspoon dried thyme
Salt and crushed pepper to taste
Fresh chives, chopped (for garnish)

Nutrition

Calories: 200, Protein: 3g, Carbohydrate: 15g, Fat: 14g

INSTRUCTIONS

1. Preheat oven to 350°F (175°C).
2. Melt butter over medium heat. Add mushroom slices and cook until tender and browned about 5 minutes.
3. In a bowl, mix cooked mushrooms, cream cheese, sour cream, and thyme until well combined. Powder it with salt and crushed pepper.
4. Spoon the mushroom and cream cheese mixture into phyllo pastry shells.
5. Arrange filled shells on a baking sheet. Bake until pastry is crisp and filling is heated through, about 10 minutes.
6. Garnish with chopped chives before serving.

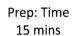

Prep: Time
15 mins

Cook Time
20 mins

Serving
4

BAKED MUSHROOM AND SPINACH PHYLLO CUPS

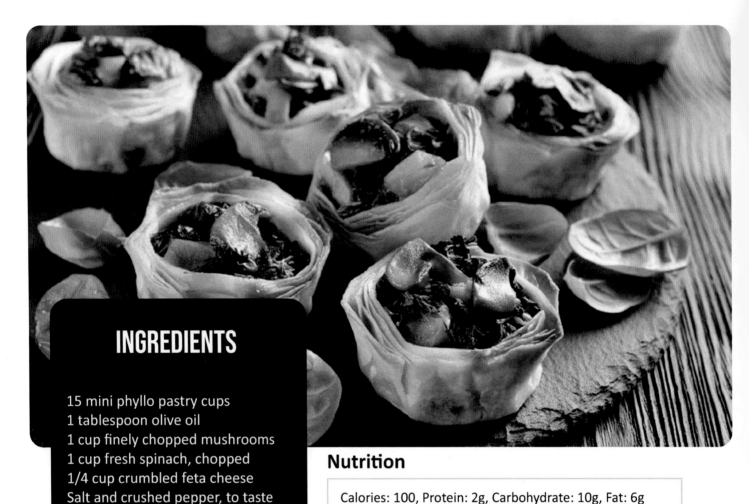

INGREDIENTS

15 mini phyllo pastry cups
1 tablespoon olive oil
1 cup finely chopped mushrooms
1 cup fresh spinach, chopped
1/4 cup crumbled feta cheese
Salt and crushed pepper, to taste
Fresh dill, chopped (for garnish)

Nutrition

Calories: 100, Protein: 2g, Carbohydrate: 10g, Fat: 6g

INSTRUCTIONS

1. Preheat oven to 375°F (190°C).
2. Heat one tbsp oil in a skillet over medium heat. Add finely chopped mushrooms and cook for five minutes until they are soft and browned.
3. Add fresh spinach and cook to wilted about 2 minutes. Remove from heat.
4. Toss in feta cheese and powder it with salt and crushed pepper.
5. Spoon the mushroom spinach mixture into the phyllo cups, filling each one.
6. Place filled cups on the parchment paper-arranged baking sheet and bake for 12-15 minutes.
7. Garnish with chopped dill before serving.

Prep: Time
20 mins

Cook Time
15 mins

Serving
6

MUSHROOM AND WALNUT PÂTÉ

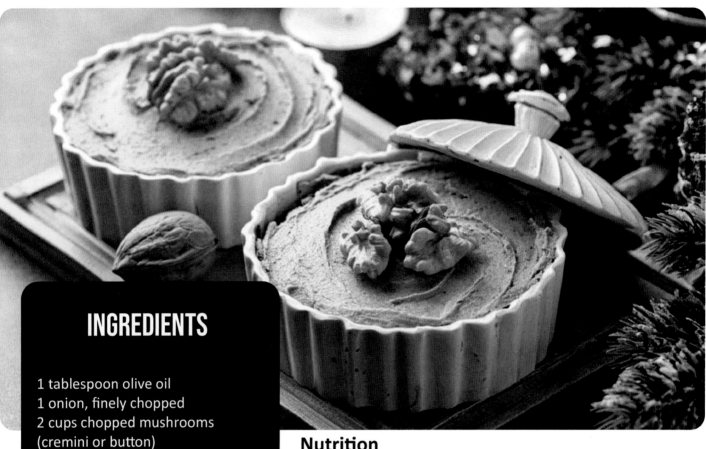

INGREDIENTS

1 tablespoon olive oil
1 onion, finely chopped
2 cups chopped mushrooms (cremini or button)
1 cup walnuts, toasted
2 cloves garlic, minced
1 tablespoon fresh thyme leaves
Salt and crushed pepper, to taste
Crackers or toasted bread for serving

Nutrition

Calories: 240, Protein: 6g, Carbohydrate: 8g, Fat: 22g

INSTRUCTIONS

1. Heat one tbsp oil in a skillet over medium heat. Add diced onion and mashed garlic, cooking until the onion is translucent, about 5 minutes.
2. Add chopped mushroom (cremini or button) and thyme and cook, for about 5 minutes.
3. Transfer the mushroom mixture to a food blender, add toasted walnuts, and blend until smooth.
4. Powder it with salt and crushed pepper to taste.
5. Serve the pâté chilled or at room temperature with crackers or toasted bread.

Prep: Time
15 mins

Cook Time
10 mins

Serving
4

MUSHROOM CEVICHE WITH AVOCADO

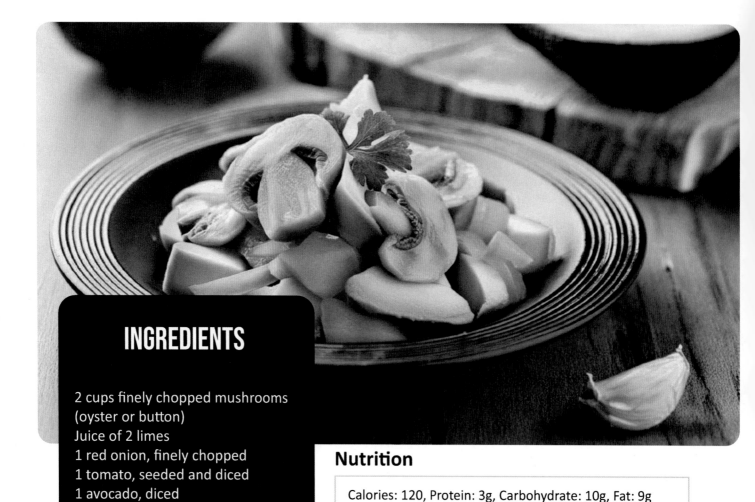

INGREDIENTS

2 cups finely chopped mushrooms
(oyster or button)
Juice of 2 limes
1 red onion, finely chopped
1 tomato, seeded and diced
1 avocado, diced
1/4 cup chopped cilantro
Salt and crushed pepper, to taste
Tortilla chips for serving

Nutrition

Calories: 120, Protein: 3g, Carbohydrate: 10g, Fat: 9g

INSTRUCTIONS

1. In a deep-bottom bowl, combine the chopped mushrooms with lime juice and marinate for about 10 minutes.
2. Add red onion, tomato, avocado, and cilantro to the mushrooms. Toss gently to combine. Powder it with salt and crushed pepper to taste.
3. Serve immediately with tortilla chips or chill to blend the flavors more thoroughly.

Prep: Time
20 mins

Cook Time
00 mins

Serving
4

MUSHROOM AND PARMESAN STUFFED JALAPEÑOS

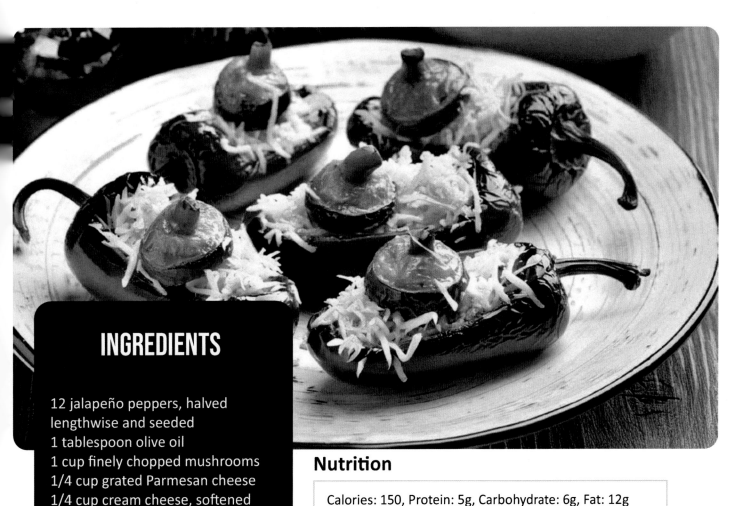

INGREDIENTS

12 jalapeño peppers, halved lengthwise and seeded
1 tablespoon olive oil
1 cup finely chopped mushrooms
1/4 cup grated Parmesan cheese
1/4 cup cream cheese, softened
1 clove garlic, minced
Salt and crushed pepper, to taste
Fresh cilantro, chopped (for garnish)

Nutrition

Calories: 150, Protein: 5g, Carbohydrate: 6g, Fat: 12g

INSTRUCTIONS

1. Preheat oven to 375°F (190°C).
2. Heat one tbsp oil in a skillet over medium heat. Add mashed garlic and mushrooms, cooking until mushrooms are soft, and all moisture has evaporated about 5-7 minutes.
3. Remove from heat and let cool slightly. Toss in Parmesan cheese and cream cheese until well combined. Powder it with salt and crushed pepper.
4. Spoon the mushroom cheese mixture into the jalapeño halves, filling each one generously.
5. Arrange stuffed jalapeños on a baking sheet and bake for 17-20 minutes.
6. Garnish with chopped cilantro before serving.

Prep: Time
15 mins

Cook Time
20 mins

Serving
4

ASIAN MUSHROOM LETTUCE WRAPS

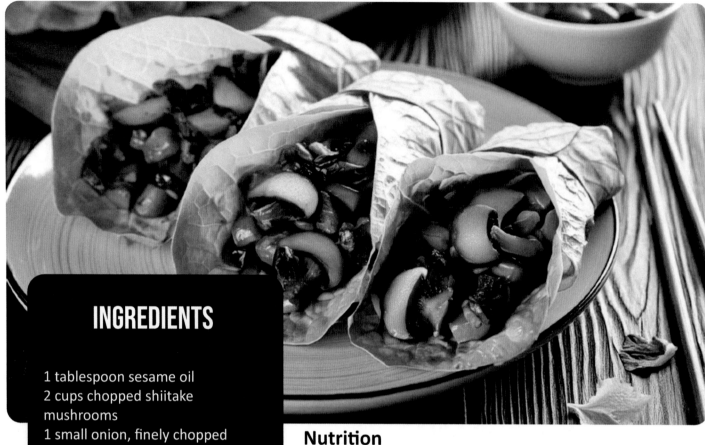

INGREDIENTS

1 tablespoon sesame oil
2 cups chopped shiitake mushrooms
1 small onion, finely chopped
2 cloves garlic, minced
1 tablespoon grated ginger
1/4 cup hoisin sauce
2 tablespoons soy sauce
1 tablespoon rice vinegar
1 head of butter lettuce, leaves separated
Fresh cilantro and chopped peanuts for garnish

Nutrition

Calories: 120, Protein: 3g, Carbohydrate: 10g, Fat: 8g

INSTRUCTIONS

1. Heat one tbsp sesame over medium heat. Add chopped onion, mashed garlic, and ginger, sautéing until the onion is translucent, about 3 minutes.
2. Add chopped shiitake mushrooms and cook until they are browned and tender, about 5-7 minutes.
3. Toss in hoisin sauce, soy sauce, and rice vinegar, cooking for two minutes until the mixture is well combined and heated through.
4. To serve, spoon the mushroom mixture into lettuce leaves. Garnish with cilantro and chopped peanuts.

Prep: Time
10 mins

Cook Time
10 mins

Serving
4

MAIN DISHES

CLASSIC MUSHROOM STROGANOFF

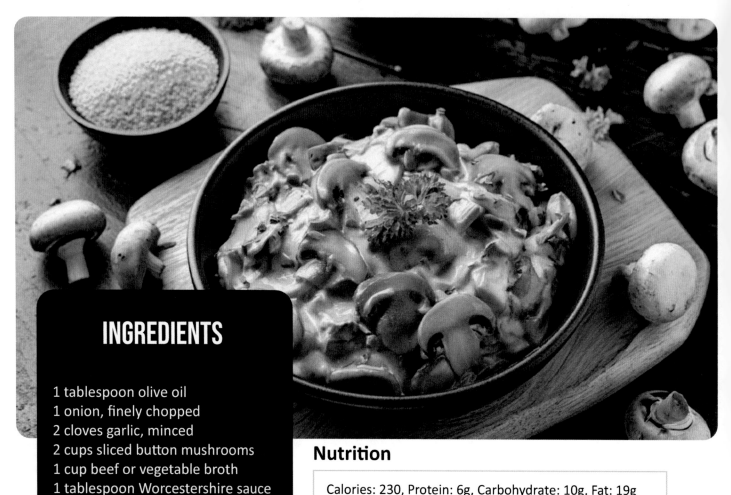

INGREDIENTS

1 tablespoon olive oil
1 onion, finely chopped
2 cloves garlic, minced
2 cups sliced button mushrooms
1 cup beef or vegetable broth
1 tablespoon Worcestershire sauce
(vegetarian version if needed)
2 teaspoons Dijon mustard
1 cup sour cream
Salt and crushed pepper, to taste
Fresh parsley, chopped (for garnish)
Cooked egg noodles for serving

Nutrition

Calories: 230, Protein: 6g, Carbohydrate: 10g, Fat: 19g

INSTRUCTIONS

1. Heat one tbsp oil in a skillet over medium heat. Add diced onion and mashed garlic, sauté until onion is translucent, for about 5 minutes.
2. Add the sliced button mushrooms and cook, about 10 minutes. Toss in the broth, Worcestershire sauce, and Dijon mustard. Take it to a simmer and cook for 5 minutes.
3. Decrease the stove heat and toss in sour cream until the sauce is smooth and heated thoroughly. Do not allow it to boil. Powder it with salt and crushed pepper.
4. Serve over cooked egg noodles garnished with chopped parsley.

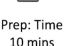

Prep: Time
10 mins

Cook Time
20 mins

Serving
4

MUSHROOM AND SPINACH LASAGNA

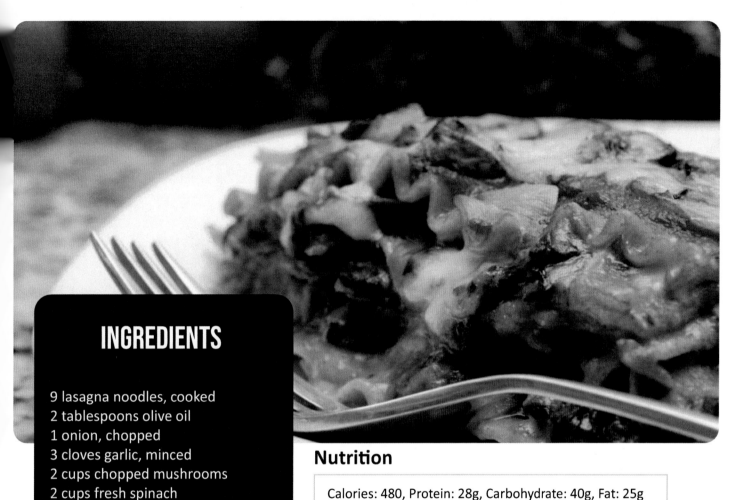

INGREDIENTS

9 lasagna noodles, cooked
2 tablespoons olive oil
1 onion, chopped
3 cloves garlic, minced
2 cups chopped mushrooms
2 cups fresh spinach
2 cups ricotta cheese
1 egg
2 cups marinara sauce
2 cups shredded mozzarella cheese
Salt and crushed pepper, to taste

Nutrition

Calories: 480, Protein: 28g, Carbohydrate: 40g, Fat: 25g

INSTRUCTIONS

1. Preheat oven to 375°F (190°C). Heat one tbsp oil in a skillet over medium heat. Add diced onion and mashed garlic, cooking until soft, about 5 minutes.
2. Add chopped mushrooms and cook until browned about 10 minutes. Toss in spinach until wilted. Remove from heat. In a bowl, mix ricotta cheese and egg. Powder it with salt and crushed pepper.
3. Layer in a 9x13 inch rectangular baking dish: Start with marinara sauce layer, then lasagna noodles, the ricotta mixture, mushroom and spinach mixture, and mozzarella cheese.
4. Repeat the layers, end with the noodle layer topped with sauce and mozzarella. Cover with foil paper and bake for thirty minutes.
5. Unfoil and bake for 15 minutes more, until cheese is golden and bubbly. Let stand for 10 minutes before serving.

Prep: Time
20 mins

Cook Time
45 mins

Serving
6

PORTOBELLO MUSHROOM STEAKS

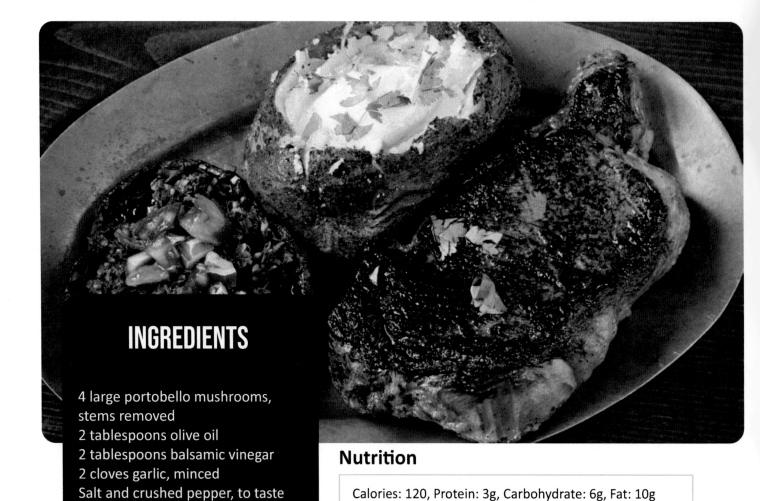

INGREDIENTS

4 large portobello mushrooms, stems removed
2 tablespoons olive oil
2 tablespoons balsamic vinegar
2 cloves garlic, minced
Salt and crushed pepper, to taste
Fresh herbs (thyme or rosemary), chopped (for garnish)

Nutrition

Calories: 120, Protein: 3g, Carbohydrate: 6g, Fat: 10g

INSTRUCTIONS

1. Preheat grill or grill pan. In a small, deep-bottom bowl, toss the olive oil with balsamic vinegar and minced garlic.
2. Brush the mushroom caps on both sides with the oil and vinegar mixture. Powder it with salt and crushed pepper.
3. Grill the mushrooms for about 5 minutes on each side until they are tender and grill marks appear. Serve hot, garnished with fresh herbs.

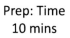

Prep: Time
10 mins

Cook Time
10 mins

Serving
4

MUSHROOM BOLOGNESE WITH PAPPARDELLE

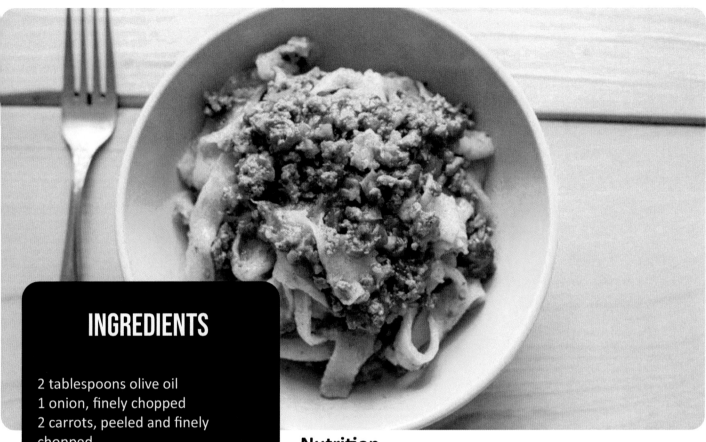

INGREDIENTS

2 tablespoons olive oil
1 onion, finely chopped
2 carrots, peeled and finely chopped
2 celery stalks, finely chopped
3 cloves garlic, minced
2 cups chopped portobello mushrooms
1 cup red wine
1 can (28 ounces) crushed tomatoes
1 teaspoon dried Italian herbs
Salt and crushed pepper, to taste
12 ounces pappardelle pasta
Fresh basil, chopped (for garnish)
Grated Parmesan cheese (for serving)

Nutrition

Calories: 480, Protein: 14g, Carbohydrate: 72g, Fat: 13g

INSTRUCTIONS

1. Heat one tbsp oil in a skillet over medium heat. Add diced onion, carrots, and celery, cooking until softened, about 10 minutes.
2. Add mashed garlic and mushrooms, cooking until mushrooms are browned, about 5 minutes. Ladle in red wine, simmering until reduced by half, about 5 minutes.
3. Add crushed tomatoes and Italian herbs. Simmer for 12-15 minutes. Powder it with salt and crushed pepper.
4. While simmering, prepare pappardelle according to the steps written on the package until al dente. Drain.
5. Toss cooked pasta with mushroom bolognese sauce.
6. Serve garnished with chopped basil and grated Parmesan cheese.

Prep: Time
15 mins

Cook Time
30 mins

Serving
4

GRILLED MUSHROOMS AND POLENTA

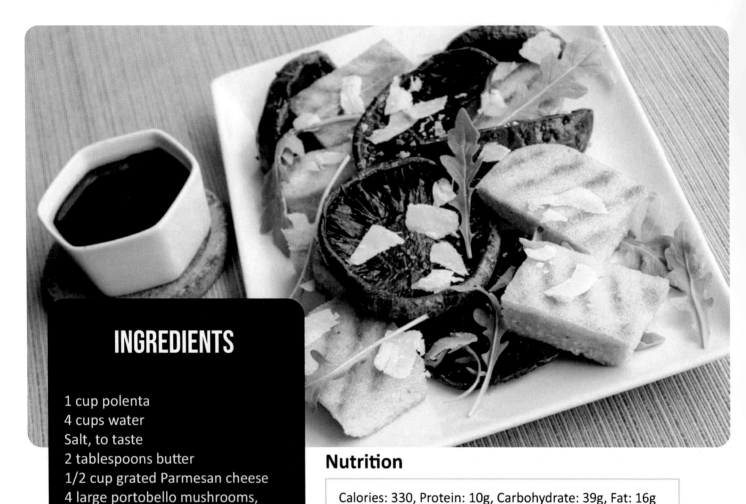

INGREDIENTS

1 cup polenta
4 cups water
Salt, to taste
2 tablespoons butter
1/2 cup grated Parmesan cheese
4 large portobello mushrooms,
cleaned and stemmed
2 tablespoons olive oil
2 cloves garlic, minced
Fresh parsley, chopped (for garnish)

Nutrition

Calories: 330, Protein: 10g, Carbohydrate: 39g, Fat: 16g

INSTRUCTIONS

1. Put a saucepan and add water to a boil. Gradually whisk in polenta and salt. Decrease the stove heat to low and cook, stirring frequently, about 15-20 minutes.
2. Toss in butter and Parmesan cheese until melted and incorporated. Keep warm. Preheat the grill to medium-high heat. Brush mushrooms with olive oil and garlic.
3. Grill mushrooms for about 5 minutes per side until tender and grill marks appear. Serve grilled mushrooms over creamy polenta. Garnish with chopped parsley.

Prep: Time
10 mins

Cook Time
20 mins

Serving
4

CREAMY MUSHROOM AND CHICKEN CASSEROLE

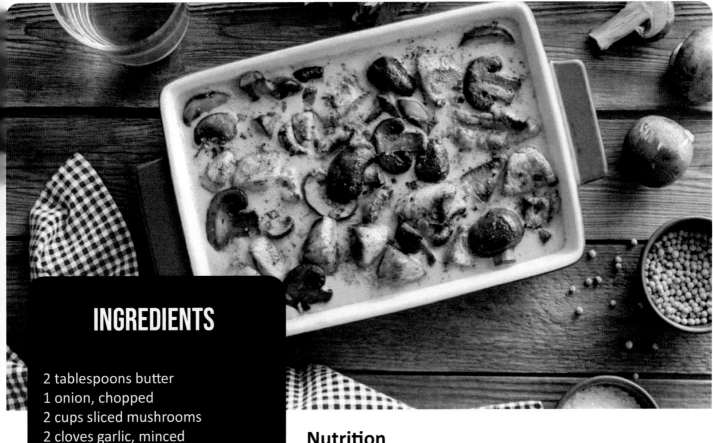

INGREDIENTS

2 tablespoons butter
1 onion, chopped
2 cups sliced mushrooms
2 cloves garlic, minced
2 cups cooked, shredded chicken
1 cup sour cream
1 can (10.75 oz weight) cream of mushroom soup
1/2 cup chicken broth
1 cup shredded cheddar cheese
1/2 cup breadcrumbs
Salt and crushed pepper, to taste

Nutrition

Calories: 370, Protein: 25g, Carbohydrate: 15g, Fat: 23g

INSTRUCTIONS

1. Preheat oven to 375°F (190°C).
2. In a skillet, melt butter. Add chopped onion, mushrooms, and mashed garlic, sautéing until softened, about 5 minutes.
3. Take the large shallow bowl, toss cooked chicken, sautéed mushrooms and onions, sour cream, cream of mushroom soup, and chicken broth. Mix well. Powder it with salt and crushed pepper.
4. Transfer the mixture to a greased 9x13-inch rectangular baking dish. Sprinkle with shredded cheddar cheese and breadcrumbs.
5. Bake for 30 minutes. Serve and enjoy.

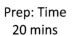

Prep: Time
20 mins

Cook Time
30 mins

Serving
6

MUSHROOM AND EGGPLANT MOUSSAKA

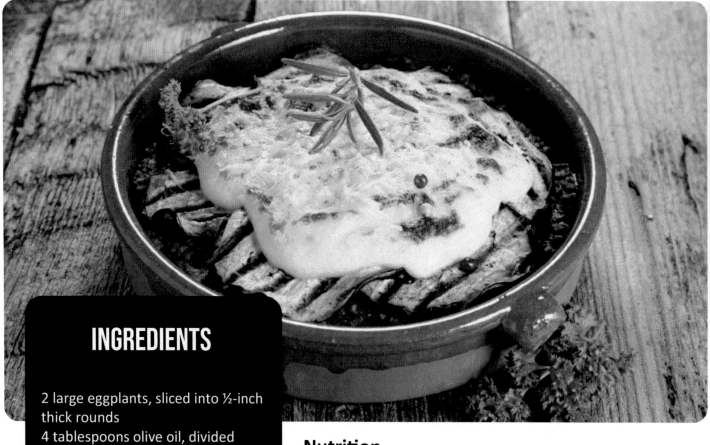

INGREDIENTS

2 large eggplants, sliced into ½-inch thick rounds
4 tablespoons olive oil, divided
1 onion, finely chopped
3 cloves garlic, minced
2 cups chopped portobello mushrooms
1 can (14 oz) crushed tomatoes
1 teaspoon dried oregano
Salt and crushed pepper, to taste
2 tablespoons all-purpose flour
2 cups milk
1/4 teaspoon nutmeg
1/2 cup grated Parmesan cheese
Fresh parsley, chopped (for garnish)

Nutrition

Calories: 290, Protein: 10g, Carbohydrate: 25g, Fat: 18g

INSTRUCTIONS

1. Preheat oven to 375°F (190°C). Brush eggplant slices with two tbsp oil and place on a baking sheet. Bake until slightly golden, about 15 minutes, turning once halfway through.
2. Heat the leftover oil in a skillet over medium heat. Add diced onion and mashed garlic, cooking until soft, about 5 minutes.
3. Add portobello mushroom and cook until they are browned and their moisture has evaporated, for about 10 minutes.
4. Toss in crushed tomatoes and oregano. Simmer for 10 minutes. Powder it with salt and crushed pepper. Set aside.
5. In a saucepan, whisk flour and two tbsp milk until smooth. Add the leftover milk and bring to a simmer, stirring constantly until the sauce thickens. Remove from heat, and toss in nutmeg and half of the Parmesan.
6. In a greased baking dish, put the eggplant layer, followed by the mushroom mixture, and then another layer of eggplant. Pour the white sauce over the top and sprinkle with the remaining Parmesan.
7. Bake for 30 minutes until the top is golden and bubbly. Garnish with chopped parsley before serving.

Prep: Time	Cook Time	Serving
30 mins	45 mins	6

MUSHROOM-STUFFED ACORN SQUASH

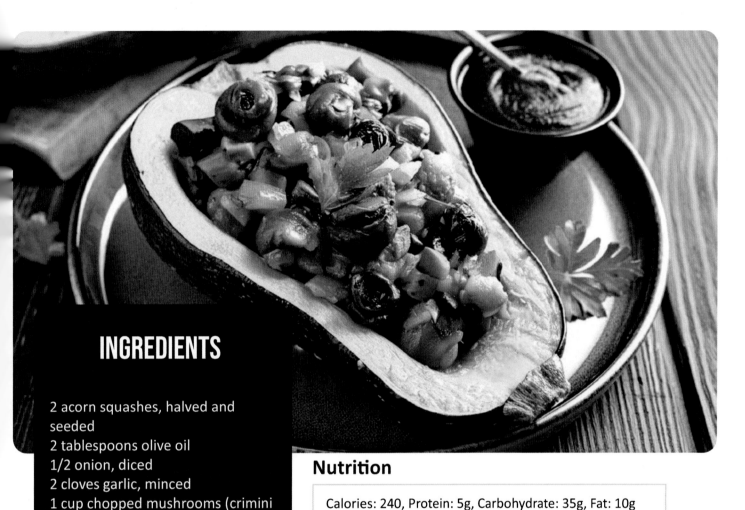

INGREDIENTS

2 acorn squashes, halved and seeded
2 tablespoons olive oil
1/2 onion, diced
2 cloves garlic, minced
1 cup chopped mushrooms (crimini or shiitake)
1/2 cup breadcrumbs
1/4 cup grated Parmesan cheese
1/4 cup dried cranberries
Salt and crushed pepper, to taste
Fresh thyme for garnish

Nutrition

Calories: 240, Protein: 5g, Carbohydrate: 35g, Fat: 10g

INSTRUCTIONS

1. Preheat oven to 375°F (190°C). Place acorn squash halves cut side up on the paper-arranged baking sheet and brush with one tbsp oil. Powder it with salt and crushed pepper. Roast until tender, about 30-35 minutes.
2. Heat the leftover oil in a skillet over medium heat. Add diced onion and mashed garlic, cooking until softened, about 5 minutes.
3. Add mushroom (any crimini or shiitake) and cook until browned about 5 minutes. Remove from heat.
4. In a deep-bottom bowl, combine the mushroom mixture, breadcrumbs, Parmesan, and cranberries. Powder it with salt and crushed pepper.
5. Spoon filling into the roasted acorn squash halves. Return to the oven and bake for 15 minutes until the topping is golden. Garnish with fresh thyme before serving.

Prep: Time
15 mins

Cook Time
50 mins

Serving
4

SPECIALTY MUSHROOMS

LION'S MANE CRAB CAKES

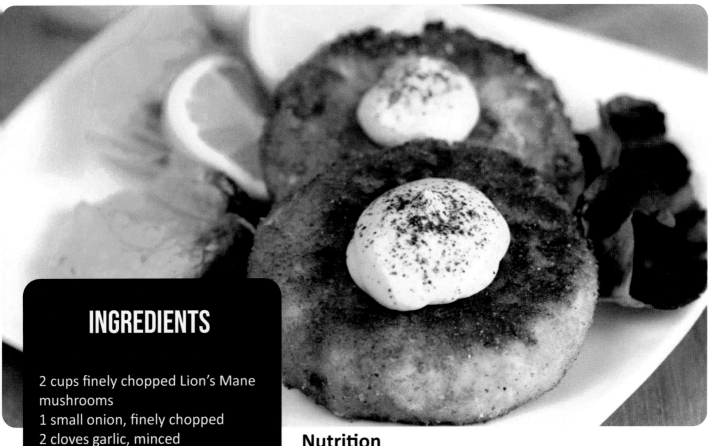

INGREDIENTS

2 cups finely chopped Lion's Mane mushrooms
1 small onion, finely chopped
2 cloves garlic, minced
1/4 cup mayonnaise
1 egg, beaten
1 teaspoon Dijon mustard
1 teaspoon Worcestershire sauce
1/2 cup breadcrumbs
1/4 cup fresh parsley, chopped
Salt and crushed pepper, to taste
2 tablespoons olive oil for frying

Nutrition

Calories: 280, Protein: 6g, Carbohydrate: 18g, Fat: 20g

INSTRUCTIONS

1. Take the large shallow bowl and mix Lion's Mane mushrooms, onion, garlic, mayonnaise, egg, Dijon mustard, Worcestershire sauce, breadcrumbs, and parsley. Add salt and crushed pepper.
2. Form the mixture into patties. Heat one tbsp oil in a skillet over medium heat. Fry the patties for about 5 minutes for one side, or until golden brown and crispy. Serve hot with tartar sauce and lemon wedges.

Prep: Time
20 mins

Cook Time
10 mins

Serving
4

SHIITAKE MUSHROOM BACON

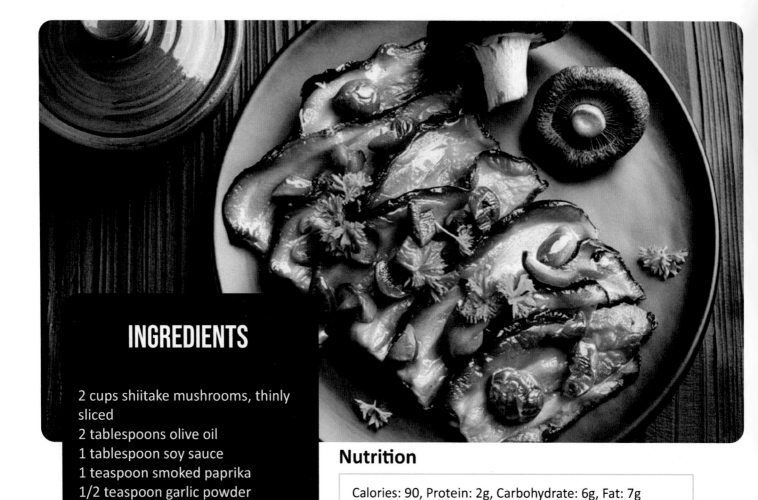

INGREDIENTS

2 cups shiitake mushrooms, thinly sliced
2 tablespoons olive oil
1 tablespoon soy sauce
1 teaspoon smoked paprika
1/2 teaspoon garlic powder
1/2 teaspoon maple syrup

Nutrition

Calories: 90, Protein: 2g, Carbohydrate: 6g, Fat: 7g

INSTRUCTIONS

1. Preheat oven to 375°F (190°C). In a deep-bottom bowl, combine olive oil, soy sauce, smoked paprika, garlic powder, and maple syrup.
2. Add shiitake slices to the bowl and toss to coat evenly. Spread the slices in one layer on a baking sheet lined with parchment paper.
3. Bake for 17-20 minutes until crisp, turning halfway through cooking. Serve as a topping on salads, in sandwiches, or as a snack.

Prep: Time
5 mins

Cook Time
20 mins

Serving
4

MAITAKE FRIED 'CHICKEN'

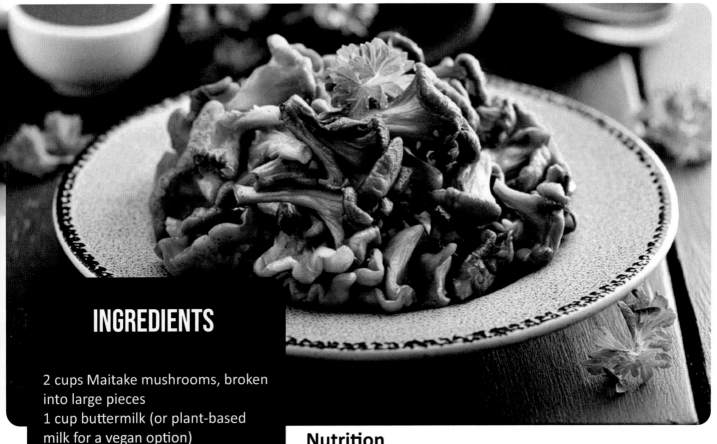

INGREDIENTS

2 cups Maitake mushrooms, broken into large pieces
1 cup buttermilk (or plant-based milk for a vegan option)
1 cup all-purpose flour
1 teaspoon garlic powder
1 teaspoon onion powder
1 teaspoon smoked paprika
Salt and crushed pepper, to taste
Vegetable oil for frying

Nutrition

Calories: 270, Protein: 6g, Carbohydrate: 28g, Fat: 15g

INSTRUCTIONS

1. Soak Maitake mushroom pieces in buttermilk for at least 10 minutes.
2. Use the other bowl and toss the flour with garlic powder, onion powder, smoked paprika, salt, and pepper.
3. Heat oil in a deep-bottom skillet over medium-high heat. Remove mushrooms from buttermilk, dredge in flour mixture, and fry for 5 minutes for one side.
4. Drain the oil on paper towels and serve hot with your choice of dipping sauce.

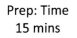

Prep: Time
15 mins

Cook Time
10 mins

Serving
4

WHITE OYSTER MUSHROOM AND BOK CHOY STIR-FRY

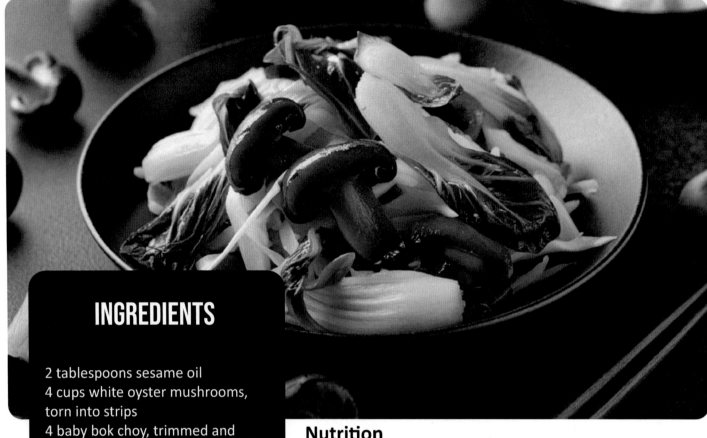

INGREDIENTS

2 tablespoons sesame oil
4 cups white oyster mushrooms, torn into strips
4 baby bok choy, trimmed and leaves separated
2 cloves garlic, minced
1 tablespoon ginger, grated
2 tablespoons soy sauce
1 tablespoon oyster sauce
1 teaspoon chili flakes (optional)
1 tablespoon sesame seeds

Nutrition

Calories: 130, Protein: 5g, Carbohydrate: 10g, Fat: 9g

INSTRUCTIONS

1. Heat two tbsp sesame oil over medium-high heat. Add white oyster mushrooms and stir-fry until they begin to brown, about 3 minutes.
2. Add mashed garlic and ginger, and stir-fry for another minute until fragrant. Add bok choy and stir-fry until the leaves wilt and the stems are tender-crisp about 3 minutes.
3. Toss in the soy sauce, oyster sauce, and chili flakes if using. Mix well to coat the vegetables and mushrooms. Sprinkle with sesame seeds before serving.

Prep: Time
10 mins

Cook Time
10 mins

Serving
4

CHESTNUT MUSHROOM BEEF STEW

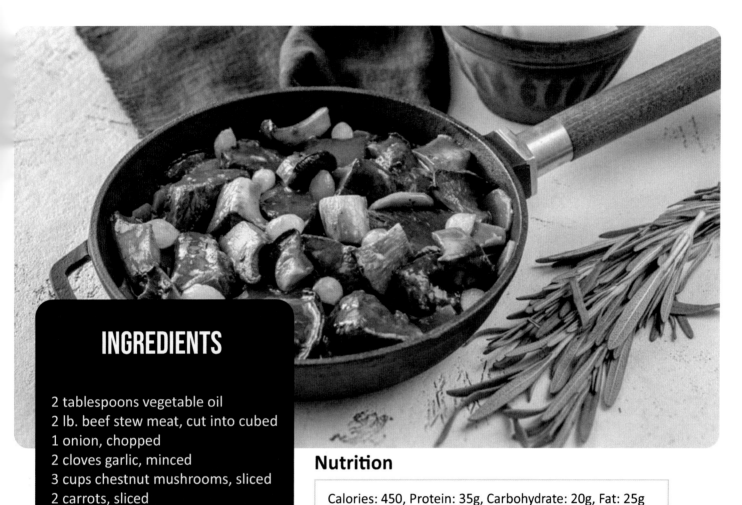

INGREDIENTS

2 tablespoons vegetable oil
2 lb. beef stew meat, cut into cubed
1 onion, chopped
2 cloves garlic, minced
3 cups chestnut mushrooms, sliced
2 carrots, sliced
2 potatoes, cubed
4 cups beef broth
1 cup red wine
1 tablespoon tomato paste
2 teaspoons thyme
Salt and crushed pepper, to taste

Nutrition

Calories: 450, Protein: 35g, Carbohydrate: 20g, Fat: 25g

INSTRUCTIONS

1. Heat oil in a deep-bottom pot over medium heat. Brown the meat cubes on all sides for about 8 minutes. Remove and set aside.
2. In the pot, add onion and mashed garlic, and cook for 5 minutes.
3. Add chestnut mushroom slices and cook until browned about 5 minutes. Return the beef to the pot. Add carrots, potatoes, beef broth, red wine, tomato paste, and thyme.
4. Take to a boil, then decrease the stove heat to a simmer. Cover and simmer for 1.5-2 hours until the beef is tender. Powder it with salt and crushed pepper. Serve hot.

Prep: Time
20 mins

Cook Time
2 hours

Serving
6

LION'S MANE MUSHROOM AND SCALLOP PASTA

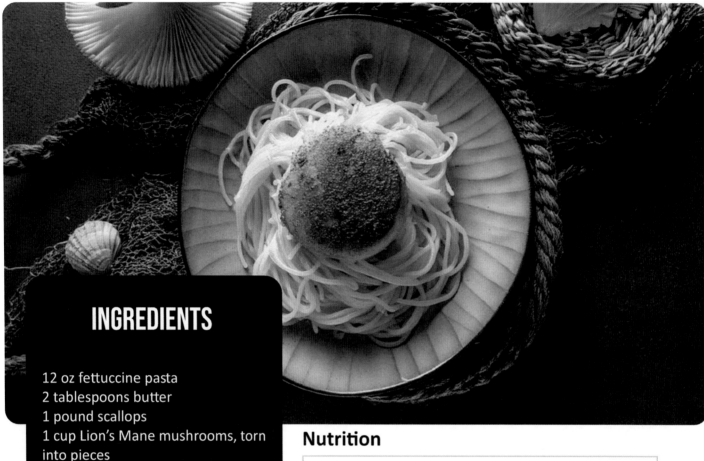

INGREDIENTS

12 oz fettuccine pasta
2 tablespoons butter
1 pound scallops
1 cup Lion's Mane mushrooms, torn into pieces
2 cloves garlic, minced
1/2 cup white wine
1 cup heavy cream
Salt and crushed pepper, to taste
Fresh parsley, chopped (for garnish)
Grated Parmesan cheese (for serving)

Nutrition

Calories: 660, Protein: 30g, Carbohydrate: 57g, Fat: 33g

INSTRUCTIONS

1. Prepare fettuccine as per the steps mentioned on the package until al dente. Drain and set aside.
2. Heat butter over medium-high heat. Add scallops and sear for 2-3 minutes for one side. Remove and set aside.
3. Use the same skillet, add Lion's Mane mushrooms, and cook until they begin to brown for about 5 minutes. Add mashed garlic and sauté for another minute until fragrant.
4. Add white wine and let it reduce by half.
5. Toss in heavy cream and bring to a simmer. Cook until the sauce get thickens texture slightly, about 5 minutes. Return scallops to the skillet. Powder it with salt and crushed pepper.
6. Toss cooked pasta in the sauce. Spread chopped parsley on top to garnish and grated Parmesan cheese.

Prep: Time
15 mins

Cook Time
20 mins

Serving
4

MAITAKE MUSHROOM AND WALNUT PESTO PIZZA

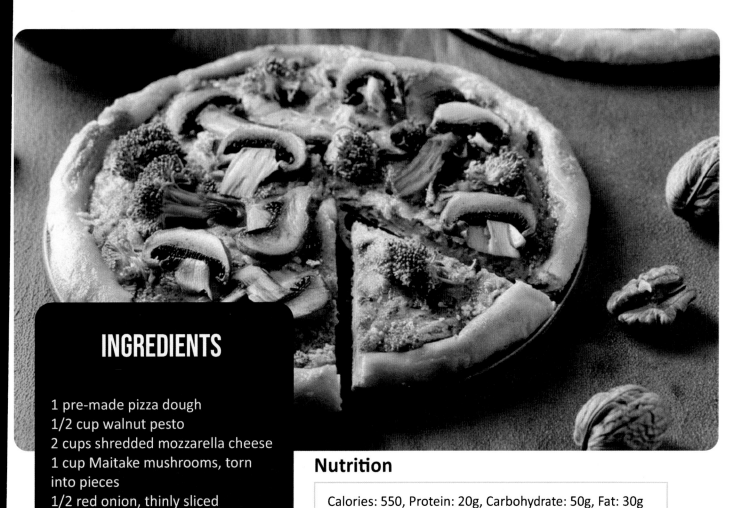

INGREDIENTS

1 pre-made pizza dough
1/2 cup walnut pesto
2 cups shredded mozzarella cheese
1 cup Maitake mushrooms, torn into pieces
1/2 red onion, thinly sliced
2 tablespoons olive oil
Salt and crushed pepper, to taste
Fresh arugula, for garnish

Nutrition

Calories: 550, Protein: 20g, Carbohydrate: 50g, Fat: 30g

INSTRUCTIONS

1. Preheat oven to 450°F (230°C). Roll out pizza dough on the smooth flour-dusted surface and shift to the paper-arranged baking sheet.
2. Spread walnut pesto evenly over the dough. Top with shredded mozzarella, Maitake mushrooms, and red onion slices.
3. Drizzle olive oil over the toppings and powder it with salt and crushed pepper.
4. Bake for 12-15 minutes until the crust turn golden and the cheese is bubbly.
5. Remove from oven and let cool for a few minutes. Garnish with fresh arugula before slicing and serving.

Prep: Time
20 mins

Cook Time
15 mins

Serving
4

CHESTNUT MUSHROOM AND GRUYÈRE TART

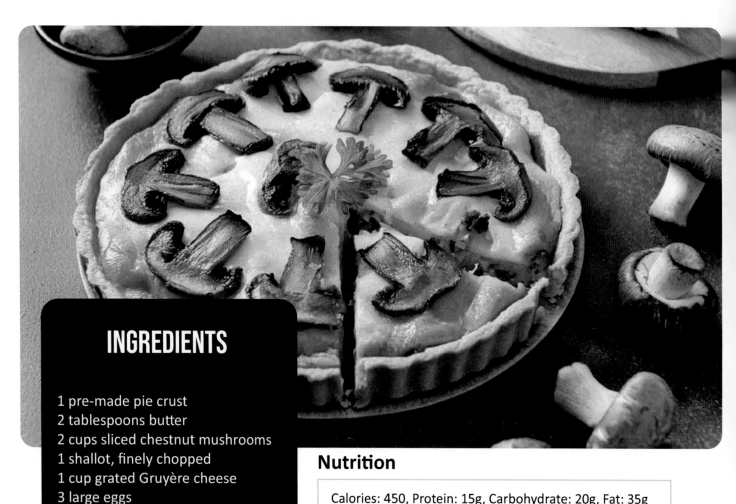

INGREDIENTS

1 pre-made pie crust
2 tablespoons butter
2 cups sliced chestnut mushrooms
1 shallot, finely chopped
1 cup grated Gruyère cheese
3 large eggs
1 cup heavy cream
Salt and crushed pepper, to taste
Fresh thyme leaves, for garnish

Nutrition

Calories: 450, Protein: 15g, Carbohydrate: 20g, Fat: 35g

INSTRUCTIONS

1. Preheat oven to 375°F (190°C). Fit pie crust into a tart pan and prick the bottom with a fork.
2. Melt butter over medium heat. Add chestnut mushrooms and shallot, sauté until mushrooms are tender and golden, for about 10 minutes.
3. Spread the mushroom mixture evenly over the pie crust. Sprinkle grated Gruyère cheese on top.
4. In a deep-bottom bowl, toss the eggs and cream. Powder it with salt and crushed pepper. Pour this mixture over the cheese and mushrooms.
5. Bake for 31-35 minutes until the filling is set and the top is lightly browned. Garnish with fresh thyme leaves. Serve warmly.

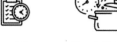

Prep: Time
25 mins

Cook Time
35 mins

Serving
6

GRILLED BLACK PEARL MUSHROOMS WITH HERB BUTTER

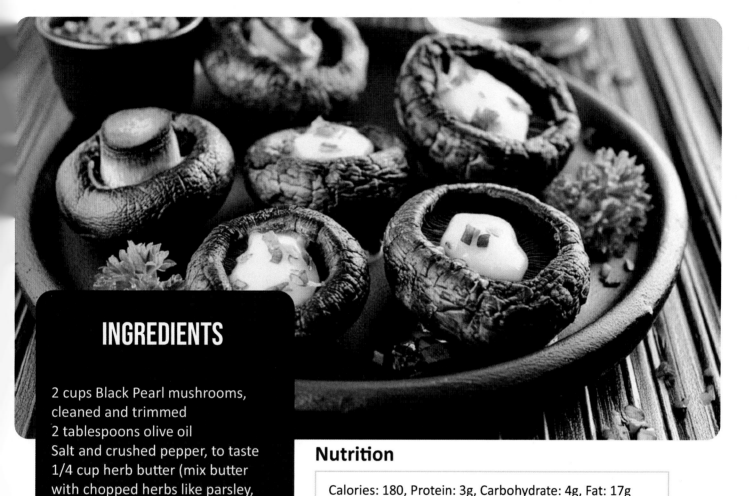

INGREDIENTS

2 cups Black Pearl mushrooms, cleaned and trimmed
2 tablespoons olive oil
Salt and crushed pepper, to taste
1/4 cup herb butter (mix butter with chopped herbs like parsley, chives, and garlic)

Nutrition

Calories: 180, Protein: 3g, Carbohydrate: 4g, Fat: 17g

INSTRUCTIONS

1. Preheat grill to medium-high heat. Toss Black Pearl mushrooms with olive oil, salt, and pepper.
2. Grill mushrooms for about 5 minutes on one side. Remove from grill and immediately toss with herb butter until mushrooms are well coated.
3. Serve immediately.

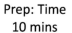

Prep: Time	Cook Time	Serving
10 mins	10 mins	4

GOLDEN OYSTER MUSHROOM CEVICHE

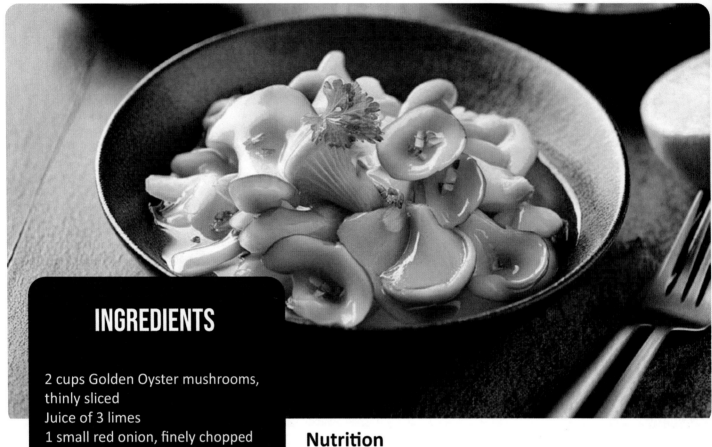

INGREDIENTS

2 cups Golden Oyster mushrooms, thinly sliced
Juice of 3 limes
1 small red onion, finely chopped
1 jalapeño, seeded and minced
1/2 cup chopped cilantro
1 avocado, diced
Salt and crushed pepper, to taste

Nutrition

Calories: 120, Protein: 2g, Carbohydrate: 10g, Fat: 9g

INSTRUCTIONS

1. In a deep-bottom bowl, combine sliced Golden Oyster mushrooms with lime juice. Let marinate for 10 minutes.
2. Add red onion, jalapeño, cilantro, and avocado to the mushrooms. Stir gently to combine. Powder with salt and crushed pepper to taste. Let the mixture sit for 10 minutes more to allow the flavors to meld.
3. Serve chilled, with tortilla chips as a light and refreshing appetizer or salad.

| Prep: Time 20 mins | Cook Time 00 mins | Serving 4 |

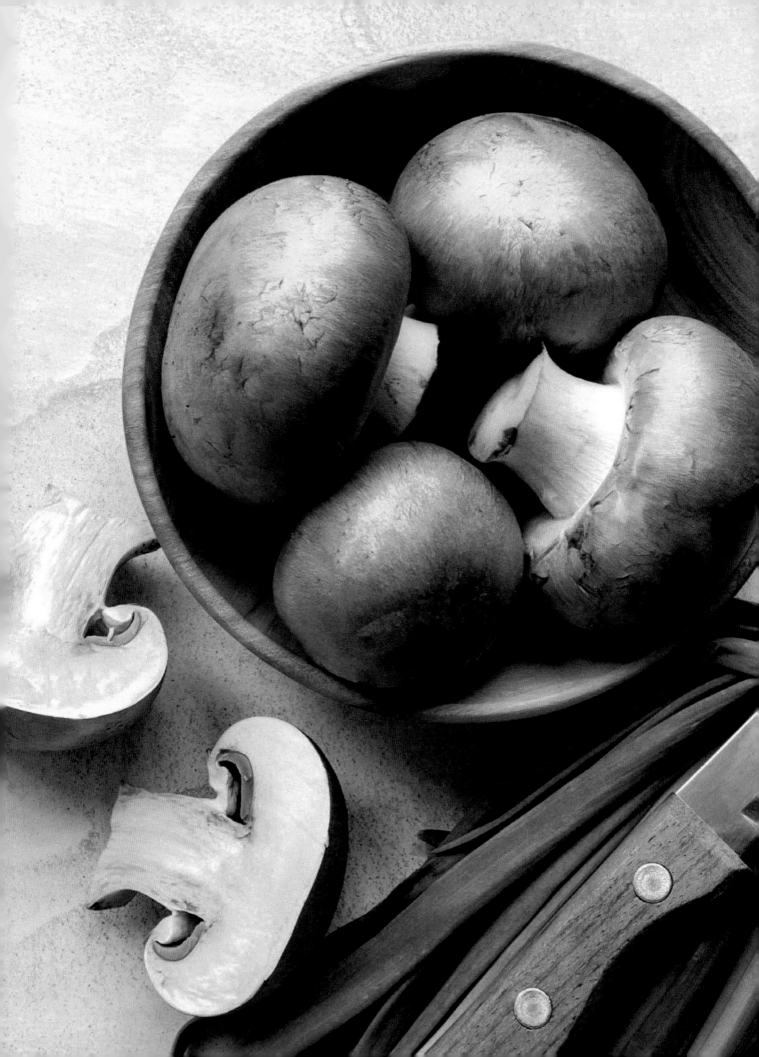

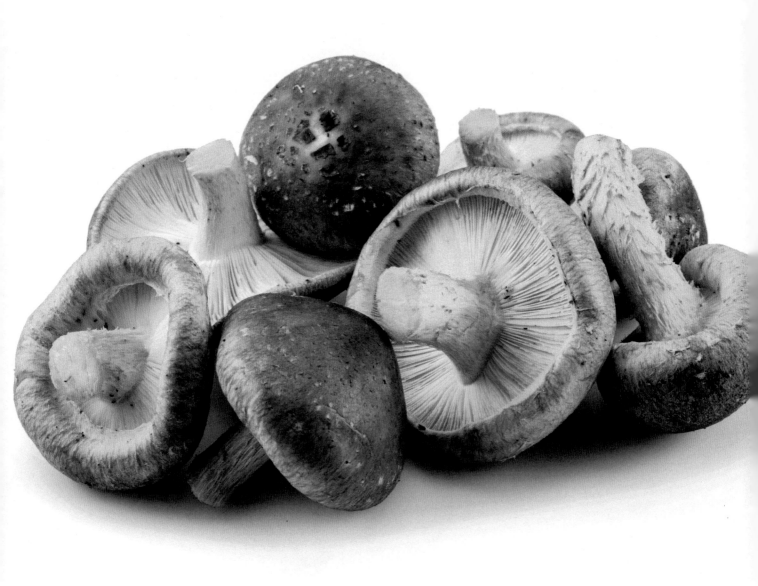